Standing Room Only

Josh Liccardi

ISBN-13: 979-8-9886153-9-2

151 Productions www.151productions.net

Printed in the United States of America.

Cover Art by: Shawn Tetreault

www.spactetotem.com

Table of Contents

To Jay....

1. Awake

Waking up wearing yesterday's clothes is not really considered an ideal way of life. Although for me it's the only way. For some reason I have found myself in this permanent situation and I am not quite sure as to when it will pass. Perhaps it will never pass and I will be stuck with the person that I have become forever. Providing nothing horribly bad happens to me along the way. I would describe my life as somewhat of a roller coaster that never actually goes up. Instead it just keeps rolling around, and many times, travels downhill with lots of small bumps and curves that follow. Getting off of this roller coaster ride will take more than an act of god – it will have to be something inside of myself that breaks this cycle of nothingness. That is what scares me the most, because changing the way that I am is not going to be the simplest task. I have tried before and failed miserably, almost instantly, but somehow I always walk away from each experience feeling better about myself.

It wasn't always like this. I actually had a great upbringing for the most part and I never really had much pain in my life at all. I can't really explain how I got into this situation, although I can explain some factors that contributed to it along the way. One thing that always bothered me, even as a child, is the fact that I never knew my father. If I was to meet him today I would most likely react in a very hateful manner towards him. This part of me has always been missing from my life. I will never understand how a person can bring a child into the world and then just leave them alone like it never even happened. This is the main reason why I have so much resentfulness towards him. I feel betrayed and I also feel as though my mother was betrayed. Being left alone at eighteen years old with a child to raise on her own must have been a turning point in her life that will last forever. Not to say that I was a burden so to speak, but just that raising a child is extremely hard, especially without the help of the partner who helped to create them. I know my father's name, but I have never seen him or talked to him. He left before I was even born and never came back or even bothered to try and help my mother in any way. My mother remarried when I was four years old and had another son. I got along great with my stepfather, but I still always felt like a part of me was missing. Over the years I have grown wiser and tried to get over the fact that my father has gone off and started a life of his own without me in it. You can only harp on things for so long before they gain too much power and start to control your life completely.

So now I find myself in a state of disarray. My surroundings would be considered odd to any normal person who was just waking up for the day. Loud obnoxious conversations can be heard from the people who drift past. The morning traffic is continuous and also deafening in its own regard. I am in the back bed part of a truck which is covered by perhaps one of the greatest inventions of all time – a truck cap. This is my girlfriend's Nissan pick up truck that I am describing, my current place of residence. We have lived together in the back of this god awful vehicle for approximately two months now. I have a small collection of blankets, comforters, and worn out pillows that line the truck bed all around to help keep warm at night. Another commodity that can be seen is my small boom box which thankfully has eight D type batteries in it. Without the pleasure of listening to music I would probably go mad, especially under these conditions. My clothing consists of mostly stolen goods that help to also support my habit. On the street new clothing is almost as good as cold hard cash. I have learned this over the years and used this currency many times for some good old fashion trading of goods.

I drop the tailgate and make my way out onto the street to start another fresh day of fighting the craving that has managed to possess my veins. Waking up is the worst part of the day because I never know what this new day will bring me. There's always a question in the back of my mind whether or not I will even get the opportunity to face the next day. Sometimes this idea doesn't sound all that bad. Many people speculate that in death there is no pain. I don't know if this is certain, but to me it makes a lot of sense. I am not religious, so the thought of an afterlife is basically out of the question. I prefer to believe in something other than commercial religion. I prefer to believe that everything around us is simply amazing in its own unique way. There doesn't necessarily need to be an explanation for everything. The thought of fate has also never made any sense to me either. Especially for someone in my shoes. If everything that we do is already planned out, than what is the point in even living, or for that matter trying to live a normal, healthy, meaningful life? This type of rationale just doesn't work with my train of thought. It is actually quite depressing if you really think about it. Of course my opinions would be thought of nothing more than the ramblings of a junkie. Maybe someday a person with much more credibility than me will step forward and speak thoughts that are similar to mine. Maybe that person will make a change that will stick and cause people to look at their own belief systems and religions. A whole nation of people will be freed from the control of church and bible study. I fear that this will never happen in my lifetime though. Instead everyone sticks to the same routine of working their nine to five jobs, and then going home to their loving families afterward just to get up the next morning only to repeat this whole cycle again. The one good thing about the way I live my life right now is the whole adventure aspect. Everyday is a new adventure with new dangers lurking behind every corner. Getting through the day requires immense problem solving skills, and revolves around me getting back to the truck for safety. I feel as though I am in a game of some sort, or even a movie. A movie that just doesn't seem to ever end. This is the life that I have chosen for myself, and it is the life that I must continue to lead. I by no means want to die, but I fear that eventually death is inevitable in the near future. A person can only go on the way that I have for so long before something terribly bad happens. I have had many scares and many close calls with such things, but nothing powerful enough to make me actually want to stop using. I have however tried countless times to give it up, only to watch myself fail miserably every time. This is extremely depressing, and makes it even harder to kick the habit.

Giving it all up may sound like an easy thing to do, but its definitely not. The average person who preaches about how bad drugs are and how people should just stop using them doesn't understand the power that these chemicals actually have. My drug of choice is none other than the evil opiate derived drug of heroin. I have tried just about everything that there is out there, with the exception of a few choice exotic drugs that are simply too hard and dangerous to get your hands on. After dabbling in all of the other choices, it seemed as though I was always on the hunt for something more. Something that made me feel like nothing else in this world ever has before. I found that something the first time I shot heroin. There was my solace. The sanctuary that I had been looking for all these years. It was like I had found a new best friend, a new reason to live so to speak. heroin became the reasoning behind everything that I did, day in and day out. My schedule completely revolved around it. A new group of friends had grown to engage in using with me. That is usually how it starts. Someone introduces their friend to this wonderful thing and then before you know it both you and your friend are shooting up all the time. Every day turns into a quest for this substance like a search for the Holy Grail or the Fountain of Youth. That is how important this drug is to us. That is how important this drug is to me.

2. School

High school was the biggest drag for me. It was all that I could do to get the hell out of there. Every day I dreamt of being anywhere but there. I hated the teachers, I hated all the rules, I hated all my classmates, and mostly I hated the classes themselves. Everything that we learned about seemed to be complete and utter bullshit. I couldn't believe that these teachers were actually getting paid enough money to own houses and lead normal lives. They didn't do anything. The only thing I learned in high school was how to weed through all of the useless shit that they claim to teach you and actually find things that would be helpful in the real world. I think that 90% of the students graduated with virtually no common sense whatsoever. This I blame solely on the education system and it's a shame when you think about it. In the "real world" common sense is perhaps your greatest asset. Most likely that's the only reason why I am still alive today.

High school is basically a big mindfuck anyways the way I see it. I never had any problems understanding the concepts that they supposedly taught, I just never completed any homework or showed up to class half of the time for that matter. Teachers don't respect kids who have a reputation for getting suspended – even if your biggest offense is getting caught smoking on campus. That was my biggest vice at the time, and still is for that matter. Why I ever picked up a cigarette in the first place is beyond me, but it's got me good now, and I mean good. I can't usually go an hour without lighting one up. That's why sometimes I'm like "yeah lets shoot up, the smokes are going to kill me anyways!"

After high school I went straight out in search of employment. At this point in my life drugs had only played a small part. I had experimented with the usual things that most high school kids do. Alcohol, weed, some mild acid, and that was about it. Things like coke and heroin had never even been offered to me. In fact it's funny how people portray schools as being this big center for drug users and drug dealers to peddle their wares all around campus. I think I got my hands on some weed twice while I was actually on the campus itself. This is one reason why the so called drug problem in this country will never be solved. People are just too fucking stupid, and have no clue as to where this stuff even comes from. As long as there is a drug, there will be people buying it and using it, that's it. It's a simple concept that doesn't take much sense to figure out. Of course if you are one of those people who graduated high school with honors or whatever you would probably think that the above statement is insane. There I go with the use of good old common sense again, stay tuned, there will be a lot of that.

In my search for employment I had trouble finding a job that I felt suited me well. Not to say that I was a lazy kid or anything, let's just say that I didn't get much pleasure out of wasting each day away stuck behind a counter taking food orders for teenagers. I would rather spend my time hiking for weeks on end in the woods, or hanging one hundred and twenty feet off of a large rock face in the middle of nowhere. These were my two only passions in this filthy world besides music. I love music with every inch of my body, although the thought of me becoming a musician left my brain at a very early age. I had no type of musical talents at all and once pursued drumming in middle school, only to become the best drummer there and be used every year in the Memorial Day march through the center of my little hometown. That was not really my idea of drumming and therefore I stopped doing it after going to high school. Maybe that wasn't the best choice in the world to make, but I have never really been known for making great choices. So with musician stardom out of my way I delved into the real things that made me feel as one. Two things that I could do almost any time were rock climbing and hiking. I simply loved it. I had just about every wonderful device and piece of rock climbing equipment that you could imagine. I spent virtually every cent on these things, and also got lots of choice pieces for birthdays and Christmas alike. These were my absolute prized possessions. I had a pretty good size group of friends that also engaged in these hiking and climbing trips with me. Sometimes we would be gone for three weeks camping out on the side of a mountain two states away. This is why I didn't have much regard for a job. Jobs prevented me from everything that I wanted to do. It also didn't make much sense to me that during the one period of time in my life where I could actually enjoy these things that I was expected to work eight hours a day; only to find myself retired at the ripe old age of sixty-five, with no ability to go rock climbing or hiking. That bothered me to no end. So instead of holding down a nice concrete steady job, I decided to be "irresponsible" and jump from job to job while scheduling things around my hiking and climbing trips.

   In the woods I felt as though there was nothing in the world that could harm me. I can't really find the logic to explain these feelings, I just always felt invincible to everything – Including my own mind. I know that every person has a certain hobby that they are extremely passionate about, but this felt like it was something even more than that. When I was camping out, or climbing over that last ledge – I finally felt as though I was alive. It's the only time in my life that I ever feel this way. That is why I crave these things so much. Smoking of course was my only enemy, sometimes I could feel my lungs burning as I got over the last hill, but that of course didn't urge me to quit – the idea alone was simply too hard to comprehend.

3. The Exchange

As I approach the faded yellow and white house I am getting very excited about where I am and what is about to happen. What most people don't understand about a heroin addiction is the complexity that it involves. Every aspect of this drug is exhilarating and contributes directly to the addiction itself. Even copping the stuff is a rush that cannot be explained. You can almost feel the effects without even having it in your hands yet. The process of using is almost ceremonial in the sense that every move made towards shooting heightens the anticipation and makes you feel dizzy. Once again, it is a feeling that cannot easily be explained.

I walk up the steps of this broken down house knowing full well who is going to answer the door and what will be exchanged. Today I have twenty dollars which will buy me a descent size bag, however it will only alleviate the next eight hours. Most people would be content for a few days with the amount that I was about to cop. I wish that held true for myself, but not anymore. When this all started, a few months ago, getting the stuff was not an easy task at all. What I'm about to do is also not considered easy. Here I am in a city where the source of just about any drug you want is close by and readily available. So why has this task not become any easier? There are many dangers involved in the process of scoring some dope in the city that I am in. Back home, about forty miles away, quality stuff is hard to find and the prices are outrageous. This has always been a problem between me and my friends who also use. The solution to this problem is right here in the city that I am currently in. The new problem is that only I and one of my other friends are brave enough to cop dope here. There are gangs lurking around every corner ready to rob you for your drugs and steal anything that they can get their hands on. I have been shot

at while running like a maniac away from these thugs that base
their whole lives on robbing people and stealing to make money.
Of course who am I to judge anybody's lifestyle? My beat up old
car had become a perfect machine to travel forty-five minutes to
our sanctuary. All of the danger involved never stopped me. It
stopped my friends like the plague. They wouldn't be caught
dead walking up to this house right now. Drug dealers are hard
people to work with; they have to keep their own safety in mind
from getting robbed, killed, or even worse – thrown in jail.
These people here know me now though. I've been a great
customer for almost a year, so of course they love it when they
see me coming. There are no names in this business however.
Just faces. Sometimes the occasional nickname is used, but that
is it. My only passport to freedom right now is my face. And the
person on the other side of that door knows full well that I will
hand over the cash, and walk away quietly with my dope. I don't
care what has to be done for me to get my hands on the shit.
Robbery, shoplifting, car jacking, even death can all be results in
this drug world. The stuff in this city is of high quality at all
times and very affordable. That was enough to make me come
here and get it.

"What you want?"

"The usual"

"Money...........damn son, that's all you got? You're gonna
be back in like a minute."

"Whatever man, peace"

That's it. Done. No problems, no bullshit, just clean
trading of goods. The minute that little packet was pressed into
the palm of my hand I felt a rush, as if I had already booted it.
It's amazing what your body and mind can do on its own. If only
I didn't have to actually shoot this shit. Maybe I will just go
around buying it up. Maybe that can be enough of a high for me.
Nope. Not this time. In fact not anytime for that matter. Nothing
is better that shooting up.

The Exchange

It is early still so hopefully there won't be any problems between here and the journey back to the truck to get high. My girlfriend is there waiting for me to get back – she wants her own little piece of the action as well. We both use like crazy. It's actually somewhat twisted and ironic if you think about how we met each other. A few months ago my mother found out that I was using and had me sectioned to a drug rehab center back home. I was there for two weeks and actually thought that I had kicked the habit for good. I didn't know at the time how wrong I was for having such thoughts. While in rehab I met her – Nikki. We hit it off right away and helped each other get through the two weeks of hell that we were enduring. Nikki had never used heroin before. She was addicted to crack and had been court ordered to rehab. She has a four year old son and lost her visitation rights because her ex-husband told the judge that she was a junkie. We decided to stick together in hopes of keeping each other clean. I got out of rehab the day before she did and had already arranged for her to meet me at my house as soon as she got out. She showed up as promised, and I haven't been back there since

"Where the fuck have you been?" Nikki shouts at me.

"Chill, it didn't take that long, would you rather go get the shit yourself?" I snap back at her.

I unbury a small wooden box, which currently houses all of my choice paraphernalia, from underneath the mound of blankets in the corner of the truck bed. Over time you tend to find the things that work best for you, and of course never let them go. I belong to a clean needle exchange a few towns over, so obtaining them has never been a problem. The really funny thing about me shooting heroin is that as a child I was deathly afraid of needles. Giving a blood sample at the doctor's office was nearly impossible, and took forever to accomplish. I used to get so worked up about the needle that my veins would collapse. My face would turn white and I would come within seconds of passing out. Needless to say, that problem is long gone. I am so good at hitting that vein now I should go into nursing and make some good money.

Opening the creaky little box is always a great sound for me. This is a sure sign that no matter what type of shit you just went through to get this dope – none of it matters. This sound screams "it is time to get high". I have a stash of small stainless steel caps that I use to cook up in. I'm not sure where I got my hands on them but they work a million times better than those damn bent spoons that you always see in the movies. Picture the cap that you usually see on a bottle of soda. That is what these things look like just without the threading. After the dope is all cooked up the fun really starts to begin. I pull it all into the needle and get ready to spike. Once I'm in the vein I pull out on the plunger a little bit, extracting some of my own blood and adding it to this wonderful mixture. Then slowly...boot it all

These feelings are indescribable. I've heard of psychologists who tried to help heroin users by actually trying it for themselves in order to get a clear idea of its effects. I have been asked many times to describe the high that I feel, but there simply aren't enough words in the English language to even come close to explaining it. It's as if someone pressed the pause button on time itself, and then after waiting a little while, started things back up again. At least that is what I am feeling while laying here in the back of this truck, high as a kite, and happy as hell.

4. Home

Things weren't always like this. I somehow managed to graduate high school, shocking the hell out of all the teachers that I ever had. I couldn't be bothered to do anything while I was there. Everything just seemed like such a waste of time, and had no actual purpose. I almost didn't graduate due to my lack of participation in gym. They were actually going to keep me from graduating because of something as irrelevant as gym. I'll never understand this concept. Well I guess none of that really matters anyways, a high school diploma doesn't get you a thing these days. Unless you want to flip burgers all your life – fuck that.

So after high school I set out to find myself a steady job. Having not been introduced to heroin yet, things seemed to be going well for the most part. I had a junky little '86 Shelby that my grandparents helped me buy. This was my trusty means of transportation. I found a job cashiering at the local supermarket – not the most ideal position but it was better than nothing. I met some interesting people while working there – a couple of individuals who you could actually have a somewhat intelligent conversation with. Things were going great for about a year or so, and then all kinds of shit started to hit the fan.

I was out late drinking one night, and ended up at this guy's house that I used to go to school with. I noticed some new people hanging out when I got there, but didn't think much of it. A short time later, however, it looked as though I was about to acquire a new friend. His name was Brad. Brad loved to party and didn't really know the meaning of the word "work". He bounced from job to job carelessly just making enough money to get him through the week until he found something else. He didn't really seem to be too concerned about the future. Brad didn't really care about anything for that matter. In many ways this made me envy his lifestyle, and attitude. I wanted the ability to not care about anything and just live life day by day taking everything in stride the way that he always did. I mean this kid would just walk out of his job if someone pissed him off enough. Just like that he would up and quit. I longed for that type of attitude and confidence. At the time, of course, I wasn't thinking about the consequences that come with that attitude. Nobody ever informs you of all the shitty decisions and mistakes you are about to make until it is too late.

So here I am hanging with Brad, wanting to be like him in so many ways, however not sure how to change my attitude. He also had quite the reputation around town for getting into trouble. Nothing too serious though, mostly misdemeanors here and there that required him to complete some bullshit community service. Brad had lost his license a few times and had been caught shoplifting on numerous occasions. It was almost as if these petty situations magnetized right in Brad's direction. It was as if he couldn't get away from making the wrong decision or breaking the law. This was the only part about him that I didn't admire quite so much. At the time I had never been in trouble with the law and didn't really want to start getting arrested.

The apartment that we are all partying at tonight belongs to another friend of mine named Dave. Dave and his fiance moved in last month and offered me the option to split the rent with them three ways. It was a situation that I couldn't really pass up. I've wanted to move closer to work anyway, and the rent is very affordable in that configuration. Even against my mother's wishes – I decided to take them up on it. My brother helped me move my small stash of belongings, and everything has been going great so far.

As I sit here, sipping on a beer, I can't help thinking to myself that there has to be something more to life than this. There has to be something more meaningful out there. Is this what I am going to do for the rest of my life? Get up - go to work every morning, come home and drink myself to sleep with my friends?

I'm not satisfied with this type of lifestyle. I have no desire to go to college, at least not at this point. High school has turned me off of seeking any kind of higher education. I know that with my diploma alone, however, I am never going to get a descent paying job. To me it is like a large double edged sword. Without a degree in something, I am basically nothing, however with a degree I am basically also nothing unless I know someone in a company that I want to work for. I've heard many stories from friends and acquaintances that actually completed college and achieved their degree. It doesn't really make anything easier – most of the time it all boils down to the interview anyway. The only edge during this process is actually knowing someone on the inside. Perhaps while growing up I chose the wrong direction to follow. Perhaps I chose incorrectly, and I will continue to do so in the future. Perhaps what I'm doing is right – I don't know yet. All of these unanswered questions constantly swim around in my head – as time goes on, I hope that I will be able to answer some of them.

5. Enlightenment

ack to work just like any other day. Here at the lovely supermarket to scan groceries for fat rich white people who can't seem to find anything better to blow their hard earned money on. Seeing the types of foods that people buy is astounding. Some of the shit that goes through my line looks almost inedible to me. Hundreds of dollars worth of complete trash gets processed by my hands alone every single shift that I work. In a lot of ways I don't see how eating this junk is any worse than taking drugs. It's just another way of poisoning your body so why not at least feel some sort of sensation while doing it? Alcohol has *become* quite acceptable in our society, as well as tobacco for that matter. What's the difference between these substances and "illegal" drugs? Nothing. The difference is that there is a lot of money to be made off of these acceptable forms of death, therefore it's perfectly ok for people to consume them - whatever.

My friend Brad decided to stop in on this particular night and come through my line with a twelve pack of Beck's.

"Hey, meet me at Dave's when you get out of here, I want to show you something." He says to me with an evil grin on his face.

"Oh yeah? What's that?" I ask.

"Trust me....you'll love it." He shoots back.

"Sure."

And that was it. That was the four sentence conversation that will in turn ruin my life. That was the grand introduction to all the bullshit that was about to come. Nobody ever really knows what they are about to get themselves into. Even if you think that you know, you actually don't. I suppose that's why we all "learn from our mistakes". So far my entire education has been based on just that – making mistakes. I tend to fuck everything up the first time, and then figure out why after the damage is already done. I wonder if there are people out there that always make the right decision. People who can always foresee the consequences of a particular decision that they are about to make. This is where I usually fail. Perhaps I just don't think that far ahead. I want to live life in the moment, and try to enjoy every second that I am here. After all life is short and I don't want to miss out on anything.

I can say confidently at this point that I don't have many regrets to speak of. I've made some horrible decisions in the past, but instantly learned from each one. I've learned some great things in this process, and wouldn't change anything that has already transpired. These little bumps in the road have just managed to make me stronger. As far as my happiness goes right now, that's another story. I am definitely not satisfied with working at a grocery store, and I am definitely not satisfied with my current financial situation. I barely earn anything right now, and never really have any extra money to throw around. I suppose I could always try to get some more hours, but that doesn't sound too appealing either.

As I left work that night I had no idea what I was about to get myself into. I thought that Brad had gotten a new CD that he wanted me to hear or something stupid like that. I got in my piece of shit car and felt an immediate wave of depression as I started it up and was reminded about all of the things that were mechanically wrong with it. I was desperately looking for something more in my life; something that held more meaning. It seemed as though you get done with high school and then struggle through life until you are old enough to retire, and then you have enough money and resources to live comfortably. It's ironic to me that freedom comes when you don't give a shit anymore - when you are more concerned about your health and well being than anything else. You finally attain ultimate freedom, but can't physically enjoy the things that always interested you. At sixty-five years old I'm probably not going to be hitting up every concert that I can get myself to. I'm probably not going to hike all over the place and find gigantic rocks to climb. That makes me believe that I actually have nothing to look forward to in the future. I want to focus all of my energy now on doing those things – while I still can. I want the system itself to be flipped around the other way – at least then it would actually make sense. I want to start my career when I'm 40 years old and have already had as much fun as possible. It's too depressing to think of myself sitting around all day long doing nothing at all. I don't ever want to get old.

I arrive at Dave's and walk inside. Brad is the only one there as Dave and his fiance have gone out for the evening. This is where I will meet my new best friend. A friend that so many people around the world already know, a friend who doesn't criticize or judge you at all, a friend who makes you feel better about yourself, at least for the time being. This friend, however, can become your enemy immediately after your very first meeting.

6.   The Law

Early morning creeps up suddenly and our almost vacant parking lot is starting to receive its first visitors. The sounds are faint as each new car pulls in and parks for the day. Work is starting for some, for people like me, it's nothing but endless hassles.

"Honey....wake up."

"What's going on?" I said sleepily.

"We have to move the truck, there are some police cars about a block away." Nikki answers frantically.

It's times like this that suck for me the most. Constantly dodging cops and moving from one place to another without getting picked up is an ongoing problem. It actually takes a lot of work to live this type of lifestyle. There are lots of things to keep in mind during the day, and especially at night. The city we're in is quite dangerous. The gangs that roam the streets are relentless in their ever growing effort to steal your dope or anything of value that you might posses. About a month ago I witnessed a very disturbing car jacking. I was walking down the street when I saw this kid come running out into the middle of the road and approach a car that was stopped at a red light. He held a gun up to the driver side window and just shot without even saying a word. He didn't even try to scare the guy out of the vehicle; he just killed him, opened the door, threw him out onto the road and stole the car. I couldn't believe it. At the time it scared the shit out of me, but I have gotten pretty used to seeing shit like that around here.

The truck has been parked in a remote parking lot all night that seemed to be a private lot of some sort for a small apartment building. We have to choose a different place to park it just about every night, because the police quickly catch onto a vehicle being in the same place over a few days time. It's risky enough parking it here seeing as how we don't have a little parking permit thing hanging from our rear view mirror like the rest of the cars here. No matter how hard we tried we couldn't find anywhere to go last night so we took our chances. We usually stick to legitimate places like grocery stores and the like, but have to constantly rotate where we go so that our truck doesn't start to become a permanent fixture. So far our luck has been very good in the last few months. We have been asked by various police officers to move out of certain restricted zones, but never had the truck searched or anything like that.

Back on the open road without any special place to go we start to scan for a new place to dock the truck for the rest of the day. By this time it is about 2:00 in the afternoon. Nikki and I were both completely sedated until about 5 minutes ago from our first fix of the day. It is now time to cop some more shit and do it all over again. Things have the potential to get ugly if we go too long without using. A few hours are really all we have in between hits. Our entire day is spent shooting up and then sleeping for a bit before shooting up again. This why holding down a job, while in the grips of this addiction, is virtually impossible. I was able to continue working for a few months when I first started using, but things quickly spiraled out of control. I didn't even use half as much as I do now. This is what happens when you use heroin on a regular basis. A tolerance is built rather quickly – the demands for more are ever present, and irresistible. Suddenly you find that the normal dose you are used to just won't cut it anymore. You have to have more. You need to have more. The vicious cycle increases from that point, and before you know it you are burning through shit like water. Your thumb aches from pushing the plunger down on the syringe too much. You can shoot up anywhere and at any given time within seconds. Your routine has been set, and perfected –

stopping it is out of the question. There is no real way to "control" a heroin addiction – it always gets worse.

"Over there by the book store."

Parking the car during the day isn't that big of a deal. Not many cops bother cruising retail stores staring at parked cars. It's only at night when the flags are raised, and these lots become a target. For now we should be fine here, as long as we keep a low profile and go about our normal routine without being spotted. This is one skill that both of us have gotten very good at.

We decide to go back to the spot together this time for more shit. It's a cold December day, but the sun is shining brightly which has made what little snow that has accumulated almost disappear. Days like this cause a wave of guilt to flow through me. I think about my old friends that I haven't spoken to at all in the past year or so. Friends that I grew up with who shared my love for the outdoors. I haven't spoken to them, but in reality – they haven't spoken to me. My life is a mess, and I have been pushed out of the group because of my drug use. We would smoke some pot once in awhile, of course, but never anything to this extent. They have all continued to lead happy lives without tainting their every thought with drugs – unlike myself. Sadly, these are the people that I want to be surrounded by, but I can't manage to keep myself together long enough for any of them to stick around. I don't blame them at all, and will forever feel guilty for breaking the ties that were once so incredibly strong. I had it all with them, but I still managed to fuck it up and throw it all away. I did my best to keep my drug use private, but was only able to keep up the facade for so long. Once things started to get out of control it was impossible to hide the facts. I've tried getting off of it – but I can't. Maybe I just don't want to be clean bad enough yet. Maybe I need to hit rock bottom really hard in order to finally wake up. I'm stuck in a hole with no rope to the top, and climbing out will kill me even if I try my absolute hardest. I have to force these thoughts out of my head as quickly as they enter, or else I'll never survive the streets. It's a constant struggle.

Back at the broken down house we make another exchange. Uneventful for the most part, but now I can't wait to shoot up because I'm feeling shitty. Ironically, using like a fiend also makes me feel shitty – it's a catch 22. I use nonetheless though, I have no other choice right now. I have no idea what is right or wrong at this point. I'll be happy again once the dope is swimming through my veins, even if it's only for 20 minutes, and that right there is enough to keep me going. It's enough to make everything worth it – no matter how shitty things get. Maybe this time when I wake up I'll feel so good about myself that I'll be able to withstand using again until mid morning. Maybe I will be able to cut back long enough so that I can eventually kick the habit for good, and get back to leading a somewhat normal life. A life that doesn't include me living in the back of a fucking pick-up truck. Tonight will be a fresh start – even if only in my head.

7. The Aftermath

I slowly begin to awake from a slumber that seemed to have lasted for weeks or even months. At first I'm not sure where I am or how I got here. I have blankets all over me and a comforter completely over my head. Before I make my journey out from underneath the covers I try to envision where I could be and orient myself to the room. Am I at home? The possibilities run though my mind as I pull back the comforter. Dave's house. On the floor. Brad is about two feet to my right in practically the same position. Then it all starts to come back to me in small pieces of memories that at first make no sense at all. I look up at the coffee table to find foil, needles, two lighters and some empty baggies. It looks as though something quite awful happened here not too long ago.

My back aches with extreme pain as I pry myself off the hardwood floor. Another wave of flashback clouds my mind as I picture Brad and myself shooting up on the couch just a few hours ago. These unclear thoughts are all I have left of the feelings that I experienced while under the influence of heroin. I have never felt this way before and I had never experienced a high like that before. Brad was right when he said that I would love it. I got up and decided to go into the kitchen to make some coffee and also to figure out what time it was. The clock on the wall reads 11:52am. I have to be to work at 5:00pm, which I am already dreading. I want to lie back down on the couch and watch TV while drifting in and out of unconsciousness. I sit down just in time for Brad to pull himself out of his coma.

"So what do you think?" He asks barely moving his lips.

"I had no idea that I was even capable of feeling that way." I replied.

"It is a feeling like none other."

"You can say that again."

The sun started to shine in through the living room windows and I could tell that this was going to be a difficult day to get through. I felt like I hadn't slept in days; however I couldn't stop thinking about the next opportunity to hook up with Brad and do it all over again. I was hooked right from the first time. It's like this drug had my name written all over it. It was finally the lift that I was looking for and the answers to all of my problems. During the first wave of euphoria I felt invincible. I felt like I had the world in the palm of my hand. For the first time ever I felt good about myself. So why wouldn't I do it again? That's the only question that needs to be asked.

At about 3:00pm I decided to take a shower and get ready for work. Brad and I had become vegetables on the couch all day, and hadn't really moved at all. When I finally got in the shower I still had no desire to do anything at all. I went off to work and got out at about midnight. I called up Dave's house and Brad answered the phone. Apparently Dave and his fiance had never even come home the night before as they were staying at their friends house and in turn wouldn't be home tonight either. Of course Brad suggested that I come over so that we could repeat the ritual that was introduced to me the night before. I promptly agreed.

On the way over to Dave's I wasn't even thinking about consequences. In fact those thoughts never even made their way into my head. Maybe that's just the type of person that I am. It seems that I am always drawn to the things in life that I cannot have or am not able to have. Usually those things are horribly bad, and have long term effects on your mind, body and soul. It's just the nature of the beast. Things that we can have are not exciting enough. If heroin was legal and everyone you knew shot up, people like me probably wouldn't even bother doing it. It's just like drinking or smoking. For some reason our society seems to think that these things are perfectly fine to buy, sell, possess and use. However we are all taught, at an early age, how horrible these two substances are to your health, but since they are legal and deemed ok, lots of people use them freely. Heroin is no different. In fact no drug is any different than smoking or drinking for that matter. This is the reasoning in my head that filters out any negative aspects to using heroin. I don't think about what could potentially happen to me – I could get killed in a car wreck right now on my way over to Dave's. I try to live life to the fullest and if something makes me feel good about myself, I am going to do it.

I will say that I am not prepared for the change of life that is going to come from using a drug such as heroin. I guess I was ignorant in thinking that this would be a habit I could control and live with for the rest of my life. I thought that I could just use it as I wanted and would be fine going a few days or even a week without getting a fix. I mean that's basically what people do with weed. You don't have to smoke weed all the time, of course it's fun, but it's not a requirement. I definitely had no idea what this was about to turn into.

So we had the entire apartment to ourselves, which didn't really matter, as we basically got to do whatever we wanted to anyways. Dave and his fiance didn't care, although I have a feeling that they don't know about Brad's heroin use. It would make things easier in the long run if they did.

As I arrived I couldn't wait to get inside and feel the rush again. This was only my second time so I still had to pay good attention to the methods that Brad used while preparing the mixture and actually getting it inside my bloodstream. I have tomorrow off so recovering will be great; I won't have to do a thing all day. My plan is to get high, lounge all day tomorrow and then pick a time next week to do it again. I hope that tonight is as good as last night was.

8. Truck Blues

So have I made it through the whole night without another hit? Not likely. I have, in fact, had another hit. This doesn't really come as a surprise to me. I have fooled myself into thinking that I was finally done with the shit more than once. So far every attempt that I have ever made has been completely unsuccessful - obviously. I have taken too much on a few accounts, and that is definitely no picnic. Unfortunately it's always when you are very close to death when you finally realize that you may have just made a mistake. These are the times that you try to get clean and stop using altogether. This has happened to me three times so far. The first step is to get yourself checked into a decent detox center where you try your hardest to kick this unbelievable habit. The following days that ensue are pure hell. There is basically no other way to describe them. The sickness comes over you like a typhoon and all you can think of to rid yourself of the immense pain is shooting up. After the ugliness of drying out is gone you are then faced with the hardest part of getting clean – staying clean. This is a challenge that greets you face to face every morning and every night. It is amazing the hold that a drug can get on a person. Eventually, depending on the type of person you are, you simply cannot take it anymore and you give in. This essentially undoes all of the pain you just went through to get to this point in the first place. That just makes you even more depressed and chances of giving it up right away again are very slim. It seems as though the drug itself just sits back and laughs at you for being so controlled by it.

It is now about 10 pm. or so and I'm feeling pretty good just coming down from our last round of usage. I need to consider moving the truck again and camping out for the night without getting busted. There is this one parking lot on the west side of this shitty town that I purposely try to avoid due to all of the gang activity that occurs there. Junkies are easy prey for local gangs who want to steal your shit. As a junkie, you aren't really in any shape to fight off six thugs, nor do you even consider it. It's better to be robbed than killed. I do fear that tonight I will have to park the truck down there and sweat the night out. If the local cops get too familiar with our vehicle I will have even more trouble on my hands. Being locked up is no fun when you're an addict. Always searching for a way to get bailed out to go and use before you lose your mind sitting in a cell all weekend. This has happened to me a few times. Mostly for being picked up on outstanding traffic violations. I believe that there are a couple of arrest warrants out for me right now for not appearing in court. I try to keep a low profile around town, and never carry identification.

I wake up my girl and move the truck to the shitty parking lot – luckily there doesn't seem to be anyone around. This can also be a bad thing though. Neighborhoods like this are usually being watched at all times by the ones who actually run things. If we can make it until sunrise everything will be fine. It's amazing how different things are when the sun goes down. The crazy people come out and have no qualms about engaging in illegal activity. I just want to get through the night without any problems and start the drug journey tomorrow as scheduled. I keep to myself and never give anyone shit, or even look people in the face half the time. You never know when someone is going to get pissed off and take something wrong. It's a very scary feeling to be held at gunpoint during a routine drug robbery. This also forces you to replace the dope you just scored. There are many variables against you out here – every day is battle.

Back to sleep for me as the truck is now safely parked and off. I climb into the truck bed and fluff up the two blankets and pillows. Pulling myself close to Nikki in order to soak up some of her body heat, I drift back asleep once again. The nights here are bitterly cold, but somehow we manage to get through them. I have actually gotten used to being cold and it doesn't bother me as much as it used to. I simply accept it as a byproduct of this type of life. When morning rolls around I can get back out there and make some moves. Steal some shit from some of the local stores and eventually score some dope for the rest of the day. At least I will be moving around a lot, which will help keep me warm throughout the day.

9. Feeling

It hits me hard. Then it pulls through me like a freight train that is stuck on its rails, but set full throttle at its fastest speed. The pause button has been pushed. Time is slowed to an almost stop. All of the energy in the world enters me through the invisible lines that are attached to every square inch of my body. For a second I have entirely disappeared. Absorbed into everything else that is....and isn't. This feeling can only be described as indescribable. Without actually experiencing it yourself, there is no possible way that one could ever even imagine its magnitude and significance. Soon time will begin again and catch up in a strange and ambiguous way. I can see around things that normally seem so benign and unimportant. A new way of thinking takes over as I try to grasp all of the differences between what I've been told, and what I am currently actually seeing. Things that normally aren't this clear are suddenly lit up and almost transparent. Like the answers were always just sitting there right in front of me waiting to be found. This is how I want to feel all the time. I can't imagine dying without ever having felt this way – I now finally feel as though there was a point to living. A glimpse into the soul this deep should not be passed over. Never again will I see things the way that I used to – through a murky filtered lens. Never again will I feel hopelessly trapped inside of someone else's great idea that I simply do not agree with or accept. Never again will I fear that there is nothing else to be found. Never again will I search for a way to fill the voids that so profoundly populate my chest.

I know that in the physical sense I am sitting on the floor against Dave's beat up brown couch, but I can't feel it. A numbness has engulfed my body which pulsates at irregular time intervals as a reminder of its presence. A cyclone of thoughts swirl through my head like watercolors being brushed lazily onto a canvas. There is no pain in this place. No worries. No cares. Just the forever stillness of my physical self that has relaxed to the consistency of putty. This is the high. This is what we all crave, and spend all of our energy constantly seeking. It has become irreplaceable. It has become everything.

I cannot completely discern whether my eyes are open or closed at various times. Sometimes I am almost certain that they are open, and then I open them to a flash of a familiar place. At other times they seem closed and I suddenly recognize the object that I have been staring at. My mind has completely taken over, causing my actual sight to be of little or no use at all. I have engaged in a journey that seems to have no real beginning or end. I decide not to question it, and enjoy the ride to its fullest extent. That is, after all, the point.

A piece of reality battles its way into my head and a bright twinge of pain shudders through my body leaving me feeling a profound sense of vulnerability. Another reminder. This is not reality. I cannot stay here, and I must return at some point. Return to the world that brings me nothing but continuous grief and despair. The idea of going back seems so utterly insane. Why we choose to live the ways that we do will forever be an unanswered question in my head. Perhaps I can handle going back, providing I know that I will always be able to return to this place. I will deal with the reality of life on a daily basis, as long as I have the option to find peace and sanctuary at my fingertips. That might be a solution that I can accept. At least that is what I will accept right now.

Groggy feeling in my limbs and my sight begins to make more sense than it did, which is telling me that I'm starting to come down. At first, panic runs through me like an electric current arcing from a broken power line. This is it. The final spiral. Flashes of memories flood my brain and I start to slowly orient myself once again. Specific details are still very fuzzy and may take some time to return, if at all. I turn my head for the first time in what seems like hours. I slowly begin scanning the room which has suddenly filled with natural light from the windows. A few minutes ago the only visible light in the room radiated from the small lamp on the corner table. Sounds of the day moving forward seep in from outside, but otherwise all is quiet in the house. Another shard of panic rips through my chest like an ice pick. Brad.

I was not alone, and this was the first time that I remembered that fact. Why can't I hear him? He should still be here, if I remember correctly – still unsure about most of my thoughts. Too much information was hitting me all at once making me feel overwhelmed and immediately exhausted. Coffee table, remote, cups, lighter, foil, CD, couch, floor, pen, lighter, soda bottle. No Brad. I decide to stand, slowly at best. Quickly relearning how to walk, I make it through to the other side of the living room almost to the entry of the hallway, when I notice the needle still hanging out of my arm. Dark red patterns surround the entry wound and race down my forearm. I pull it out and touch the dried encrusted blood amazed at its plentiful amount. Weird.

I had originally hoped that last nights experience was going to be as good as the night before. And it absolutely was, even exceedingly so. It had been every bit as wonderful and perfect, but somehow even better than the first time. Everything had been so beautiful, right up until this very moment. I continued toward the hallway and immediately noticed Brad, face down in the middle of the floor. Still fully dressed from the night before, clearly there was a problem. Ten million thoughts all rush through my head at once rendering me frozen and helpless for a moment. Then the panic takes over as I start racing toward Brad in a feeble sort of way. Right before I am close enough to lift his head I notice the pool of vomit next to him. Fuck. I lift him up in a frenzy realizing the urgency and rush toward the door. I'm not even completely sure what to do, but I don't have many choices at this point if I want Brad to live. In the car and off we go to the hospital. Desperately trying to avoid an accident I can feel my heart thrashing out of my chest. Fuck, fuck, fuck. There is no sufficient preparation for a race against time itself.

10.   Shopping

I hadn't remembered a dream in a very long time. But this morning I woke up with very vivid details etched into my mind. At first I was excited, because I used to have great dreams all the time, and always remembered them in the morning. I'm sure that my recent inability is somehow related to the coma-like state I am usually in when sleeping, due to habitual drug use. This morning however, was different, because nothing else had changed – but I remembered.

My dream had jumped around to various places, and I was left with detailed images from each of the scenes. At one point I was surrounded by water, an ocean I think, and there was no place to swim to. No land, no boat, not even a random buoy. I was not in any clear danger except for being stranded in this endless body of water. I would swim and swim, but never get anywhere. This seemed like a sensible dream for me to be having at this time. The metaphor is clear, and spot on. The next flash took me to a battlefield of all things. I was running around in what appeared to be army fatigues and I was armed with a small ill-powered handgun. Just as I came across the enemy and lifted my gun to shoot I was shot in the neck by someone on the opposing side. Flash to me sitting in a luxury hotel room wearing a white cotton robe and sipping on a glass of water. This one made no sense to me whatsoever. I had no agenda in this scene other than keeping my water from spilling. That was my main goal at all times. It was very, very important that I did not spill one drop of water from my glass. Ironically that wasn't the odd part. The odd part was that I had no idea why I was doing this, or why on earth it was so very important to protect. Whatever. Flash, flash, flash. I am rock climbing, having a blast. Scaling my way up the face of a rock with little or no effort at all. Every overhang is easily overcome, as I move with the swiftness of a spider. I get all the way to the top in what seems like record time. Everything is wonderful, beautiful and perfect. The only strange thing is that nobody is on top waiting for me, I am completely alone, and apparently have come here all by myself, which seems unlikely. That was the last thing before I woke up.

At least now I have some interesting things to ponder during the day if I get the chance to feel a few minutes of boredom. Right now I have other things on my mind, more immediate needs. My girl is out still, and is in what looks like a very uncomfortable sleeping position. I climb out silently making sure I have what I need to get things done as quickly as possible. I am broke. I'm pretty much always broke, but right now I literally have nothing. In order to get a fix I need to come up with some currency. These days can be very daunting. It can go any number of ways, with only one way being an acceptable outcome. That is, of course, for everything to go right, or as right as it can, to provide a somewhat speedy delivery of dope. I would like to stress speedy. It isn't going to take long for my girl, and myself, to start really feeling the physical effects of the craving. My goal today is to score within the next few hours in order to quench the thirst that is just beginning to burn. I would really like to avoid becoming a stark raving mad lunatic, walking the streets hopelessly all night, becoming an easy target for local authorities. That is the last thing that I need right now. I already have a couple warrants floating out there – no need to draw unnecessary attention to myself. I must concentrate on this at all times. All they need is a reason, doesn't matter how much merit it has, there just has to be a reason.

I am walking to a shopping center that is around the corner from the truck about two blocks away. I purposefully make sure that the truck itself is nowhere near any place that I am planning on lifting some shit from. Any association would take the whole thing down. One big giant sinking ship. The truck is where we live, permanently. I know that sounds completely crazy, but I have accepted the situation I am in right now, and therefore choose the truck over the cement any day of the week. Without it many things would be extremely difficult. I need to treat it with respect and do whatever I can to protect its existence so that it can be there for me as much as possible. After my girl, the truck is second on the scale of importance – heroin obviously being the first on all of my scales.

This particular plaza is a bit run down, but not so much so that it has extensive security crawling around its grounds. In fact, this plaza is extra special because it has no security at all. Once you start living this lifestyle you start to get tips from others who are basically doing the same thing that you are. Sometimes it's for alcohol, sometimes crack, regardless, it's the same exact process. These tips are heavily guarded, however, because too much noise brings the cops around, and that ruins it for everyone. Every spot that gets blown is one less potential source of income on the map. That's how we look at it anyway. And with the invention of the video camera already spoiling enough fun on its own, it makes you actually work to avoid working entirely. I find some ironic humor in that somewhere – it makes me feel like I'm not that lazy after all.

Inside a department store filled with semi name brand clothing, I find myself over at the men's department browsing through the jeans. Jeans for some reason are guaranteed cash on the streets. Most places that actually have jeans which are sought after come equipped with those wonderful ink tag devices which explode if you try to get them off. There are, of course, people out there who have made deals with the right people and have actually acquired the proper tools to remove these devices. It's usually easy enough to find them, because they charge for their services. Sometimes it's not worth going through all the risk though of getting the really good jeans. I have found that it is just as easy to lift many pair of the slightly less profitable jeans at once, and essentially have the same pay out after. This also eliminates an extra step in the process of scoring. That's my goal today.

There is a technique that I use for department stores like these. It involves use of the dressing room, and wearing entirely too much clothing. It's a pretty simple illusion that really only works about half of the time. Most places have become very observant in a nonchalant sort of way so as to better catch a thief at work. They pretend that they aren't watching, but they have mentally recorded your every move. They also have a pretty good idea of who to watch as soon as a potential suspect walks into the store. It's always a game of cat and mouse. I start to slowly roll up a few pairs of smaller sized jeans and tuck them down the legs of a larger pair that is on the rack folded up. This particular method can be a bit sloppy; however it works, especially in stores like these. I take the folded pair with the newly constructed bundle inside and make my way to the dressing rooms, which are completely unsupervised. I'm in. The door is shut and locked. We're halfway there. As quickly as I can, but without making any noise I rip off my pants and start taking the hidden jeans out of the larger folded pair. Inside are three pairs all incrementing in size and all larger than what actually fits me. I start with the smallest and layer the other two over that one. I am now wearing three pairs of brand new jeans, and I still have to put my original pants back on. The benefits to being little can sometimes be very profitable. I wear pants that are much too big for me all the time for exactly this purpose, and for lifting other various items as well. I walk out of the dressing room with the folded pair of jeans in my hand and neatly return them to their rack. Nobody seems to be paying any special attention to me whatsoever – this might go off without a hitch after all. After poking around for about 10 more minutes so that it doesn't look like I just walked in off the street and stole a bunch of jeans in the dressing room, I head for the door. Anxiety used to hit me like a battering ram when it was time to make the exit. It doesn't at all now. It's still there, but very muted and watered down in comparison to how it used to be. Act normal. Walk steady. There is no law that states upon entering a store you must buy something. Naturally I open up the door and walk back out into the cold morning air. This time things went as planned, if there was going to be a problem I would not have gotten this far, without running that is. If they had figured me out I would have been stopped before getting outside, the golden rule is to keep them in the store until the cops show up to deal with it. I've been through that. I'm sure I'll go through it again in the future as well – occupational hazard.

There's an underpass about two blocks from here where I'll change back into one pair of jeans and organize my three new pairs that should turn into about 50 bucks. As brisk as it is out, I feel somewhat warm inside, phase one of the day has gone exceptionally well, and I can feel the corners of my mouth straining to let a smile escape. I feel pretty good about the next few steps as well, but you never know what is going to happen when you are dealing with people like this. What you knew yesterday could be completely useless knowledge today. Bad information could get you killed in an instant. Always ready and observing everything are the keys to survival. In the end, that's all you are doing anyways – surviving.

The underpass is empty today, well at this moment, which makes me happy – less bullshit to deal with. There are a few people who frequent this place quite often. Most of them are completely harmless, but there are, of course, always exceptions to the rule. When you really look at things it's not the best group of people to be around, so logically problems arise. The cops tend to stay clear of here for the most part. They make their presence known by periodically driving by and lazily shining their spotlight toward the entrance of the underpass, but rarely ever actually approach it. Sometimes the city turns its head allowing some of the riff raff to just be – providing they are nowhere near anybody else. The "don't ask, don't tell" policy isn't only effective in the army. The homeless don't ever really bother anybody, well they bother people, but not in a violent way at least. This is why the underpass gets a free ride for the most part, the police figure that they are all congregated out of the way and not causing harm to anyone, so why bother.

Using the privacy of the underpass I change out of my stolen goods and get things back in order. One stop shopping would bring me back to my usual spot, however I won't get as much dope because they won't pay as much for the pants. This is the safest route though; turning the jeans into cash requires some interaction with undesirables. In keeping with the luck of the day, I decide not to push it too much this time and settle for whatever I can get back at the usual spot. With the three pairs it should be at least enough for us to get through the night, and hopefully by then Nikki's parents will have hooked us up with another wire transfer. This has been our last line of actual income, but even that supply has been starting to dwindle.

I walk up to the dilapidated house once again, pants shoved underneath one of my arms. The exchange happens with such fluidity it was almost as if they were waiting for me to show up with the stolen goods. Weird – I am definitely not complaining. In a flash the jeans are gone, and replaced by two foil packets in the palm of my hand. My blood boils and shoots through my body with such exhilaration I can actually feel it move through my veins. This wave of relief, followed by intense anticipation, is almost just as good as the high itself. The ritual has begun, and just like the very first time, the feeling is indescribable. Happily I start making my way back to the truck, taking an unusual course to get there, so that no associations can be made between my direction and the truck itself. I can't wait to get there. I need to feel the feeling. I need to build my impenetrable fortress and hide in it for as long as I can. I need to let go of all the things that suck right up to this very moment -

and just be. That's all I ever want, and I don't think that it's too much to ask for.

Finally I am at the truck; all is perfect – and it's time. My girl will be happy because of the score, hopefully she is still asleep, and wasn't just sitting here all paranoid and anxious. I open the hatch and there she is, still passed out amongst the stash of blankets. That's good. I climb in and get ready to take care of business. Good times are here again.

11. Disaster

Dragging Brad in by his shoulders I can see people staring out of the windows at the emergency room. Nobody jumping up to help, of course, but everyone's curiosity peaked to the fullest. Just like a bad car crash that you can't keep your eyes off of. One person has been kind enough to run to the front door and hold it open for me, but other than that everyone stays in their seats. I drag him to the triage nurse who takes her time opening the window, obviously having personal issues with Brad's "ailment". Bitch. I hate people. A nurse shot through the doors displaying a lot more compassion and helped me quickly get Brad onto a gurney. Wheeling him out of the waiting room I explain to the nurse that I found him in his apartment with a needle. She shoots me a loaded look and yells some medical jargon to the surrounding nurses. The gurney was docked and one of the nurses ran over with a needle. She stuck it into Brad's arm and slammed the plunger down. Ten seconds later Brad's torso shot straight up on the gurney as he took in a large gasp of air as if breathing for the first time. My heart rate immediately started to return to normal, as soon as I realized that Brad was alive. Most of the nurses in the room were making disapproving faces and were eager to go on to the next "emergency".

We both felt it would be best if I took off. Brad is very resourceful and will find his way back to the house, or find someone else to get him. They are going to send in a counselor for a psychiatric evaluation to determine whether or not Brad has a problem. Me being there wouldn't help and would probably just make them all the more suspicious. Brad has gone through this process before at other hospitals. I was not privy to this information until right now. He knows how to answer and how to look in order to get released in a timely manner and get back out doing whatever drugs he wants. So I took off.

Brad had overdosed. He told me the broken story from his side that explained how we got here. Everything had actually gone as planned last night like I originally had thought. Brad has a higher tolerance than I do when it comes to heroin because he has been using it longer. You build up a tolerance very quickly and need to start using more in order to feel the same effects that you are so very used to. The stuff we used last night just happened to be a tiny bit stronger than usual – this is one danger that is almost impossible to avoid. As the morning hours crept up Brad decided it was time for another hit. I was still clearly high as kite when he came to this decision so he fixed himself up a shot and proceeded to indulge. Brad cooked up an amount that normally would have been fine for his system, but since he already had some of this extra strong batch swimming in his veins, it was just enough to put him over the edge. He booted it, walked toward the kitchen and collapsed in the hallway. Another hour or so and Brad would have been dead if I hadn't gotten him to the hospital when I did.

I glanced at the clock in my car which was off by two hours. After getting my brain to do the simple math I discovered that it was 1:00pm. Up until this very moment I literally had no concept of the time and would have guessed that it was 6:00am. I was planning on going back to Dave's to get some sleep as I had the night off at work. The drive back was much different than the rush to the hospital a few hours before. It felt surreal to be driving at a normal rate of speed. This took a bit of adjusting to get used to as the feeling was unexpected. Although the urge to get high washed through me, I had pretty much no desire to use at all. This had been a rough morning, and a rough aftermath to last night. I wanted the drug without all of these risks and potential dangers. I wanted to be able to feel that way without being worried about going too far or losing someone in the process. I wanted to be happy.

Dave and his fiance had still not returned home, which was good because I had some cleaning to do. The living room was cluttered with all types of paraphernalia that desperately needed to be hidden away. It looked like a pack of wolves had gotten ripped in here last night with no regard to anything else in the room. Couch cushions were dislodged and almost touching the floor. A lamp had been knocked over completely, but was still shining brightly. It seemed as though needles were everywhere. The odd thing about this scene is that I had no recollection of even moving from the floor – let alone partaking in any of its madness. Perhaps I was wrong. Perhaps I had been all over the room as the evidence clearly showed, and the illusion of me sitting on the floor up against the couch was all in my head. Perhaps my time line was off and I had completely forgotten about everything up until I landed against the couch on the floor. Who knows?

Carefully picking up needles and foil wrappings I decide which items will be useful in the future and what needs to be disposed of discreetly. As I begin to walk down the hall toward the kitchen I am reminded of the puke on the floor, and the awful smell that it has left in the house. Damn. Hopefully there's some Lysol or something floating around that I can spray everywhere, I'll just tell Dave that I got sick if either of them notice. The last thing that I want to do is sop up someone else's vomit, but it would seem that at this moment I have no choice. I'm not dealing well with the whole "no choice" thing, but that seems to be happening a lot today.

Now that everything is acceptable in the house it's time to get some rest. Recovering from last night and this morning may take a considerable amount of sleep, so I prepare myself. As I lie down on the bed and surround myself with blankets, the most uncontrollable urge smacks me in the face. Shit. I roll over trying to ignore it; maybe it will take some time before it hits me again. Panic shoots through me, which brings on another urge immediately. This is not something that I had prepared for. I guess this is what people describe as withdrawal. So soon? This is not good. I stashed everything that I deemed useful for future use in a black backpack that I always use for things of importance. I tear at the zippers frantically as the urge is so strong now that my skin feels as though it is peeling back from my fingertips. I cooked last night with Brad's help, and can easily manage it on my own. I prepare the mixture and tear a filter off of one of my smokes. Swirling a small piece of the white fiber around in the lovely elixir, I suck some up into the syringe. Not too much, we don't want a repeat of last night, and especially while I'm sitting here all alone. My veins are already jumping out of my skin with anticipation, waiting to be punctured and alleviated. One tight little pinch and I'm in. One small draw back on the plunger turns the dose red with my blood. Now the moment that I've been waiting for – One, two, three……

12. Capture

A loud hissing sound pulls me out of a stupor. For a minute or so I just sit there listening to it, not registering whether or not it is even real or just in my head. Nikki is slumped over herself in the corner of the truck half covered by blankets and completely comatose. Then it hits me. Our tires have been slashed. The truck is leveling itself slowly as each tire loses more and more air – I can feel us getting closer and closer to the ground. This is really going to put a damper on things. I don't actually hear anyone outside of the truck so I must have completely slept through the initial slashing. It must have just recently occurred because there is still significant air leaking out of the tires. I have also deduced, with the way that the truck is leveling, that all four tires have indeed been slashed. Immediately money flashes through my mind. Money that neither of us have to get this fixed, and if we do get it fixed that's a substantial amount of dope that we don't get to purchase or use. Fuck.

Nikki's parents are the type that will bail her out at pretty much any cost. I have never really understood their mentality, but I'll take it. They seem to be quite accustomed to her ways and put on a good front that they show to the world. They don't fully accept that she has a problem, or that I am with her also feeding this problem. They like to think that she is simply going through some rough times, which require their monetary assistance once in a while. The other thing that doesn't help is the fact that they have massive amounts of disposable income. Nikki's father owns a very substantial car dealership and has made loads of money from it. Her mother doesn't work and just gets to enjoy life however she likes, and what her father actually does can't really be considered work either. All that being said – for some reason they have no issue shooting us a large sum of money every few weeks. Nikki gets her mother on the phone and whines about this and that until a sufficient amount is agreed upon, and then we wait for the wire. So there is somewhat of a solution for what has just happened, but we still have the issue of fewer drugs. This is not good.

I climb out of the truck and inspect the damage. Sure enough someone has plunged a knife into the sidewall of every single crappy tire that the truck is sitting on. So that's four new tires with labor, and that's assuming there's a way to drive this thing on its rims to a nearby shop as to avoid a flatbed charge. That's also assuming that all of this happens within 24 hours so that the cops aren't swarming all over the truck getting it towed to their impound lot. One more big bag of problems dropped into my lap – how perfect. I also need more dope. Where to begin?

My girl is awake, time to break the news to her and get her on the task of spinning a web for the parents so they can get some cash to us in a timely manner. After I'm done explaining our new dilemma to her it's off to go score again. This time I am going to avoid stealing, and instead call in a favor. I have been putting this off for some time because I don't expect things to go very well. I ran some shit for this guy a few weeks ago who I've known pretty well for the last year or so. I started coming down here with my car, back when I actually had one, to score for myself, Brad, and whoever else was down at the time. The dope down here is really good, and less expensive. I was one of the only people in our group that would stick my neck out and come get it. Most of the places to score here are not nice places to be, even if you are an experienced junkie. After you come to a place like this long enough certain people start to know you. That can be a good thing, but usually it's a very bad thing. These aren't the types of people that you really want to get to know you. They are bad people, who will throw you under the bus without even blinking. Everyone is in it for themselves ultimately, and favors are not just handed out – you have to earn them.

A few weeks ago this guy that I've bought shit from a million times before in the past, asked me to make a pretty substantial sized delivery for him. I asked no questions, kept my head down and moved what he asked me to move. If it had been anybody else I would have immediately declined the task, but I do have a small thread of trust for this person and weighed the options appropriately. He told me he'd hook me up next time I needed a fix, and I believed him.   He's never let me down before and has never given me a reason to doubt his intentions, so I decide that today is the day to give it a whirl. One free ride to deal with the truck issue, and then we can get back on course tomorrow. I grab my hoodie and set out on foot – once again

This side of the city is desolate and filled with the likes of me. Families that just couldn't make it have been surrounded by drug dealers and prostitution. The houses are barely standing up on their own, and the yards are littered with broken toys and other junk. It's really a sad state of affairs. Chain link fences line most of the yards giving the false sense of protection from the junkies who roam the streets. Some of the windows have bars on them, some have boards, and some are clear as a bell with no protection at all. These are the houses that should really be avoided. If someone has decided to not display their fear of the outside world, there's usually a pretty good reason for it. Sometimes that reason is two 95lb Rottweilers and three men all holding illegal, unnumbered AK-47's. These people see no reason to have any obstructions attached to their windows. These people are the ones that I have come here to see today.

I walk up the broken stone walkway to the front door with my hands out of my pockets and in plain sight. I know that I am being watched and want to make it very clear that I mean no harm whatsoever. The lackeys that control the firepower are not usually the sharpest people and do best at taking orders while observing the obvious. Staring at the door I knock on it three times, and not too hard. A slider quickly opens up.

"Business?" A stern voice asks.

"John" I answer calmly.

The slider shuts with a large click and the locks begin to loosen their grip on the door frame. The door opens as I am welcomed inside. The living room of the house has been converted into a large office of sorts. A huge mahogany desk divides the room into essentially two halves. My half, and his half. The two dogs flank the large desk and are obediently sitting, waiting. Flanking the dogs are two very large men both holding their automatic assault rifles across their chests. The door shuts behind me and I am ushered to a seat in front of the desk by the other gigantic man who answered the door. The man who sits at the desk I know only as John. Always have. I'm certain that's not his real name, but that has always been his name to me, and I see no reason to ask questions. He is a businessman, not usually dealing with the likes of me, but we met under strange circumstances about a year ago and he seemed to take a liking to me. This could be considered bad, but so far there has never been a problem.

"What can I do for you?" John asked.

"Looking for the kickback on that drop a few weeks ago" I state with controlled confidence.

"Ahh yes, you took care of me well, I never did get to thank you properly. Take this as a token of my gratitude." John flicks a medium sized foil packet over the top of his desk toward me. It's a pretty good score for just making a drop. This is something that I could really get used to. This particular bundle feels like it will keep us going for a few days. What a relief.

"Thank you" I utter back.

"Let me know if your services will be available in the future. There will always be some work here for you if you like".

"Thanks again" I say. And slowly stand up to leave. I can feel the big hulking guy at my back as I walk toward the door. I step outside and the door shuts behind me with force. I can feel eyes all over me as I walk down the stone pathway toward the street. Everyone knows what goes on in John's house. Everyone also knows that most likely I have shit on me. This makes me an easy target. I have to get off of this street as quickly as possible and in a very inconspicuous manner. Without drawing attention to myself I cut through a field that is attached to a broken down park and disappears into a mass of trees. I turn to face the field in order to keep an eye on things and light a smoke. This has already been quite a morning, but things seem to be looking up. At least the big score will buy me some time on looking for cash. That's always a good thing. Now I just have to deal with getting the truck fixed quickly, and making the next logical step.

Time to start moving. I cut through the small patch of woods and end up facing the rear of a convenience store. Nobody is there so I step out into the parking lot and start making my way toward the front of the store. Just as I get passed the side of the store I bump right into a group of four guys standing by the corner of the building. All four of them stop talking and move into a line essentially blocking my way. Each one has that addiction ridden glaze in their eyes. Tattered clothes and bulky jackets. One of them tosses a bottle of shitty cheap beer to their right and it smashes on the ground. I'm about to get jumped. Robbed. Beat.

In this instant my only thought is on the dope. They're going to get it. They know from how I look and from what direction I came in that I'm holding. They also know that I'm holding something good, nobody comes down here for anything less than good. In this instant there is absolutely no way to protect it and that has become my biggest concern. Deep breath as they all advance toward me – I'm not going down without causing my own damage.

I smash my right palm into the face of the largest one who was coming toward my left. I figured a move like this might take out the biggest bruiser and catch the rest of them off guard for a moment. That's all I got though – a moment. The big guy that I hit went down instantly with a burst of blood spewing out of him. I must have broken his nose, which was exactly my goal. The other three had me detained immediately as I took hits starting at my chest. Once I was sufficiently beaten into a harmless state one guy went through my pockets and scored the dope in an instant. That was my fault for not putting it somewhere safer while I was in the small patch of woods. Fuck. I wasn't expecting what happened next however. Being nailed in the face with the butt of a 9mm doesn't feel very good at all. I was seconds away from losing consciousness as I felt my boots being removed along with my hoodie.

The taste of blood in my mouth is starting to become sickening as I feel my bruised stomach churning inside of me. I can't tell if anything on my body is broken because my head hurts beyond comprehension. My glasses were busted in two during the attack, which also really sucks. I can't see for shit without them, it's actually going to be difficult to find the truck now. I have another pair of shoes in the truck, but still that's one more asset of mine gone. And I loved that fucking hoodie. If not for the dope the hoodie would upset me the most. I can tell that all of my teeth are still there, and intact, as I spit blood out of my mouth. My face and head took the most of it.

I focus on getting back to the truck before I freeze to death, its cold out and I am wearing a t-shirt and an old baggy pair of pants. I hobble down the street still trying to look inconspicuous so that nobody tries to get me to a hospital. I'd be picked up in an instant by the cops, and who know what would happen to Nikki. Stand up straight and walk normal. It really doesn't help that I have blood all over the front of my shirt. At least I'm not far from the parking lot where the truck is, I just have to make it a few more minutes like this. Just then a cruiser turns onto the road from the intersection in front of me; I turn my head to pretend that I am just leisurely walking down the sidewalk. I can hear the engine getting closer and closer to me as he makes his way down the street. I take a quick peek out of the corner of my eye and notice that he's coming right for me with all of his lights flashing. I stop dead as he pulls up onto the sidewalk in front of me and jumps out of the car – gun drawn. I put my hand behind my head and drop to my knees. A single drop of blood slides down the side of my face and stains the concrete below.

13. Work

The next few days at work are daunting, and long. The clock seems to take a sick pleasure in moving only in five minute increments. The calculated beep from my register doesn't help my vegetative, robot-like state either. None of my customers have faces. They have been reduced to simple numbers. Totals to be exact. $38.52, $51.23, $10.15, $109.80, $64.11. Unless forced otherwise – this is the only time I speak. I want out. I want to run screaming from the building while tearing all of my clothes off. I want every person in here to start yelling at the top of their lungs all at the same time until all of the windows shatter. I feel like a prisoner. Like a lab rat running on his wheel – never having the ability to reach a destination. I feel like I'm dead. I've discovered that the worst thing about heroin is all of the time that you have to endure when you are not on it. Being tossed back into the real world simply doesn't seem right anymore. In my opinion it never really felt right in the first place, but now I can barely even tolerate it.

Beep, Beep, Beep. Five more minutes pass. I feel like I'm losing my mind in this place. Brad got out this afternoon. He was released from the rehab unit deemed fit to rejoin society. I have no idea how he managed to pull it off – even after his explanation. For some reason he has a knack for weaseling his way out of almost anything. The kid should have been an actor apparently. All I could think of was "wasted talent" when he told his almost unbelievable stories of deceit. You would swear that he actually believed the lie that he was telling – I suppose that's what made him so convincing. Regardless he was able to convince three different counselors that he has no chemical dependencies whatsoever, and that his "experimental" use of heroin landed him in the ER. So they let him go against protocol. I have already witnessed him slam a syringe in his arm 16 minutes after he got to the house. I know that it was 16 minutes exactly, because I was playing a little game with myself in my head. I wanted to know exactly how long he'd be able to make it before getting high. I was banking on 10 minutes tops – he surprised me.

Tonight is going to be uneventful. Or at least that's the initial plan. Brad and I are of course planning on shooting up when I get out of work. This time however, there is going to be some extra caution in place. No getting up in the middle of the night and cooking up a lethal dose of dope to leave someone on the floor lying in their own vomit. We are going to do our best to keep things a little bit safer. Apparently we got quite carried away last time somewhat trashing the living room. I still have no recollection of this except for standing on the couch laughing and screaming something inaudible to Brad. All of the rest of the details were completely new to me as Brad recapped the night. None of these things were going to go on tonight – if we could help it.

Five minutes. I am snapped out of my daydream as a lady hands me her ecologically friendly reusable bags to use on her order. Five cents comes off of her total for each reusable bag that she brought in with her. She has two bags. That's ten cents. Wow. She is also one of those people who want all of her groceries to fit inside just these two bags. After each one is packed full and right below the point of overflowing, she hoists them over the back of my register and is finally on her way. The next "number" steps up in front of me eager to have her groceries scanned and bagged. This process continues to go on and on like this. Each transaction only takes on average about two minutes unless the "number" has a particularly large order and than maybe you are looking at five minutes tops – which is where my friend, the clock, comes in - tick, tick, ticking away at nothingness. My break time has finally arrived. I get 15 minutes to do what I please with. I find myself running to the door while still fighting my way inside of my hoodie. Before the outer door opens my smoke is lit. I cannot afford to waste any of this time.

Standing outside by the pay phone I begin to contemplate building a better life for myself. I have no ambition or drive to better my education. So that plan is completely out of the picture. I need to get myself on a career path that actually interests me. Something outdoors and less structured. Something that might make a difference in the grand scheme of things. My contribution to society is a shitty one, with no real purpose and no real outcome. A monkey could perform my job, and probably even better that I can on most days. The only thing that I would ask for in a profession is to be interested in the content of the work. I'll never understand why this seems to be such an unreasonable request to make. I can confidently say that none of my current formal education has prepared me for anything in the real world. Another reason why I see no point in attending college, simply just to waste money, and time that I'd much rather be doing something enjoyable with.

I still have no plan. Oh well. Tomorrow is another day. One of these days the most perfect idea is going to fall right in my lap – I know it. How's that for naivety? Walking back into the shithole store I can't bear to look at any of my co-workers. They all seem so complacent and perfectly deceased. Perfectly willing to wait idly by and never actually get anywhere. Just like the lab rat on his wheel. Spin, spin, spin. Fuck that. I really have to get out of here. Head down, I shuffle back to my register ready to endure the remaining two hours of my shift. This is the longest stretch. If I still have arms when I leave this place tonight it will be a miracle – as that will mean that I was able to refrain from gnawing them off with my teeth. Beep, Beep, Beep. $92.78, $145.65, $23.76, $12.42. Five minutes pass. I die a tiny bit every time I peek at the clock and it's still not time to go. My tattered corpse will be all that's left of me when I finally get the opportunity to drive away from this terrible place tonight.

14. Inside

The backseat of a police car has barely enough room to be functional. I already know this, as I have had the pleasure of riding in them many times before. My knees are all but sticking into my chest as I sit sideways behind the passenger seat of the cruiser. My hands are cuffed behind my back and moving at all is an act in futility. I have never been busted for anything too bad, in my opinion at least. Never for committing a crime against another actual person or for intentionally causing anyone harm. Stealing. Possession. Those are the two big ones. The arresting officer, who is taking my on my free ride to the police station has been so kind to inform me of why I was picked up this lovely morning. After using excessive force during the arrest itself, he has decided to have a little chat with me during this short ride.

Apparently it really is a small world after all. Either that or I just happen to have some of the worst shit luck on the planet. I have definitely not ruled out the second possibility. The owner of the convenience store, where I recently had my ass handed to me, was who called the cops. It just so happens that this store owner also knows some people that work at the department store where I performed my most recent act of shoplifting. All of the store owners in the area have been giving each other physical descriptions of people they believe are ripping them off. They are all looking out for each other, just like we all do on some level. Even though I had gotten away with my most recent thievery, after I left the store, they were apparently able to put all the pieces together. The police had already gotten a call from them the day before with my description. I was recognized by the convenience store owner as well, which is more than likely the reason why he decided to call the police in the first place. It wasn't because I was beaten within a few inches of my life and robbed. It was to help aid in cleaning up the streets. Or more importantly, to protect his business from people like me.

I basically just walked into a gigantic trap with every step that I took this morning, right from climbing out of the truck. The only blessing in disguise was the beating itself. My dope had been jacked – one less possession charge for me. The police officer actually seemed agitated when he discovered that I had nothing at all on my person. Even after knowing that I had just been jumped, and had the shit kicked out of me, he was eager to see what kinds of goodies he could find. There were some really bad things to think about though. I haven't had a fix since last night. It will be afternoon soon and the withdrawal is going to begin – unbearable at first and then increasing to levels of incomprehension. There is no way around this. With my record, even as small as it is, there is no reason for them to let me go before attending the arraignment. And they won't. The problem is this: it's Friday morning. I am going to be here all weekend. Two days of intense sickness is sure to follow. And then court sometime on Monday. Then back to the streets. I am going to have to be wheeled out of here. It's going to be that bad. I am trying really hard to suppress the anger that I am feeling right now, because that is just going to bring everything on even faster. Stay calm. You can do this.

We arrive at the police station. I am dragged into a room with a large counter type desk in it for processing. After another search through all of my clothes is performed, everything is thrown into a small manila envelope and shoved into a cubby behind the desk. Contents of my envelope are – lighter, smokes, two keys, a piece of paper filled with numbers, a gold hoop earring (which I was forced to remove), and my glasses (in two pieces). Mug shot. This one must look terrible given that I am a bloodied mess. I wish there was a way to get your mug shots later; I'd love to hang them all up somewhere. Finally I get to be alone as I am led to my holding cell. I walk in and the barred door shuts behind me with a mechanical click. My cell has a metal toilet in one corner and a metal bed sticking out of the concrete wall across from it. I sit on the bed. What else is there to do really? The feeling of helplessness is overwhelming and must be dealt with immediately or every single minute in this place is going to be horrific. I try to focus on all of the ramblings that have been etched into the walls and on the bed itself.

After about an hour or so I start to get anxious as the sickness slowly starts creeping up behind me. I can feel it licking away at my back trying to take hold for good. I have to do everything in my power to prevent its consumption of my mind for as long as possible. Once it takes over - I'm finished. I will be permanently attached to that disgusting toilet in the corner. I will be a mess. Not to mention the arraignment itself. How will I be able to keep it together in a courtroom? The formalities are so stupid. I don't get it. And I am not going to try to.

Random dates and initials are littered throughout the cell. Some people feel the need to leave thier mark here apparently. As if it is important for the next person who enters to know they were here. I sit and ponder the relevance of this. I come up with nothing. Perhaps it was just a tool to pass the time and nothing else. That I can certainly understand. "Go fuck yourself" is scratched into the center of the metal bed. This is easily the best advice I've been given all day – wish I could partake. There seems to be about 8 holding cells if I had to guess. I can't see any of them right now, but when the cop was bringing me to mine I did a quick count. I can hear someone rustling around about three cells down or so, but other than that there isn't anything to hear. It is enormously quiet. I suppose for some people this is a pretty effective form of torture all on its own. It doesn't really bother me at all for some reason.

The guy down the hall starts bellowing loudly right at the same time that my stomach decides to start dancing furiously inside of me. The sickness is starting to take hold, and listening to the idiot down the hall doesn't help. I curl up into a ball on the metal bed and try to concentrate on more positive thoughts. Music, an open field in the middle of nowhere, a giant rock face itching to be conquered. Holding steady I try not to let the sickness get too much of a foothold. It is going to happen anyways, I have no way to stop it. But the longer I can fend it off the better. It's not like I have anything more productive to do. The bellowing from the other cell has started to turn into actual words being shouted. "Water". "Give me some fucking water". I am guessing that he's going through some type of withdrawal as well. It wouldn't surprise me in the least; this city is filled with junkies almost everywhere you look. It's the perfect hub for good, strong, affordable drugs. It's a utopia for people like me.

My eyes have been closed for what seems like hours even though I am certain only minutes have passed. This is going to be a very long couple of days. I am, however, bound and determined not to let my concentration break. I can't even hear the man anymore. He's still yelling – I can feel it, but I can't hear any of it. The mind is extremely powerful, and when pushed beyond normal use, can perform miraculous things. I have managed to project myself completely outside of this cell, escaping the inevitable sickness and disallowing myself to become depressed. Soon enough Nikki will start to worry about my safety. She will either assume that something went horribly wrong and I'm lying in a ditch somewhere dead, or the more obvious – I got picked up. This has happened in the past, and it has happened to her as well while I was left behind trying to figure everything out. Depending on who saw what went down this morning, word might actually get to her if she goes looking for me. Things work like that around here. I just really hope she doesn't venture too far out trying to find the answer; she's tough as nails but still very fragile in many ways.

I am woken up from my daydream when I feel a bead of sweat drip off my forehead and onto my cheek. Every bone in my body is starting to ache uncontrollably, partly from the beating, partly from the withdrawal. I could really use a hospital bed for all of this, but apparently my injuries don't seem serious enough to these people to warrant that. I wish that I had been shot. Then I could be in a hospital bed hopped up on meds and most likely sleeping through most of the withdrawal. Police officers would be taking guard at my room, but still it would be a million times better than this. I was injured just enough to be in extreme constant pain, but not enough to justify an escorted trip to the hospital. This current situation couldn't really get much worse, especially since it's only Friday.

The sweat is a byproduct of the sickness growing stronger with every second that ticks off. My shirt is starting to become soaked through as the blood stains begin taking on a new, third shade of red. Soon I will be shaking and freezing cold. After that it's all over. I will be a pile of flesh on the floor writhing about and throwing up bile from my vacant stomach. If I get through this without dying I might consider grabbing Nikki and finally getting the fuck out of here once and for all. Go back home and try to start some sort of life that makes sense again. I'm not sure if that's even possible at this point considering all of the choices I have already made to get me here. I'll worry about the logistics after I get through this. It is time to concentrate. There is much to fear about the next 48 hours. Minute after minute of torturous events will fill the rest of my time in this place.

15. Road Trip

Brad and I are in my car and cruising down the highway. My battery powered boom box on the backseat emitting a constant array of music. Driving in silence is completely out of the question and listening to the radio is even worse. We are going to score. This will be my first time going to this particular city for this reason. We are going to a place that everyone back home frequents often, mostly for shopping needs. Just a mere few blocks away from the tourist attractions lurk perhaps the largest drug network in the state.

I feel a small twinge of nervousness as we round the last corner and stop in front of a large abandoned building that resembles an old warehouse. This quickly passes as I remind myself that Brad has done this many times before, and will have my back throughout the entire process. I am being introduced to this process so we can expand our inventory options. Since I actually possess a vehicle, the two hour round trip adventure can be performed anytime, providing that there is gas in the tank. The grade of heroin here is perfect and much more affordable than back home. The same goes for the blow, which can be purchased here and used as a source of income. This place sells both.

We approach the steps of the desolate building and make our way through the first set of doors. There is nobody here guarding anything, you are completely on your own. Bums are hanging around outside and inside. Junkies are lining the walls every few feet with nowhere else to go, and in hopes of getting enough cash to score a hit. They sit here all day long hoping someone like Brad or I will have some sympathy and hook them up with a bit of cash. They have completely given up and aren't even out on the streets making moves of their own. It's a sad thing to witness. The lighting is almost non-existent inside the building. Hallway after hallway is littered with birds and abandoned cats that have decided to call this place into their home. The cats have aided in the stinging stench that emits throughout the building. Water drips erratically from somewhere and is very loud as we walk down each long dark hall. At the heart of the building is a door with a small wooden shelf built into it at eye level. Above the shelf is small cutout that obviously slides open. This is where the business is conducted.

Brad approaches the window and knocks once on the shelf. The cutout slides open immediately and a disheveled looking face peers out at us. Brad flashes one index finger in front of the opening and plops down a folded up wad of cash. A descent sized square package replaces the cash – it's wrapped in foil and otherwise non-descriptive. This is the blow we'll peddle back home to make some extra cash with. Brad then flashes what looks like a sideways peace sign with his hand, and produces a larger wad of cash on the shelf. This is replaced with an even larger packet wrapped in brown paper and adorned with a red stamped image of a scorpion. This is the dealer's way of branding their particular strain. The scorpion is good. The guy behind the cutout is not the actual dealer – just another worker for the enterprise. The scorpion brand heroin gets distributed to guys like this who set up shop in various places around the city to sell, sell, sell as much as they can before getting busted and moving their operation elsewhere. The actual dealer himself is very hard to get to and too smart to get caught. His whereabouts are unknown to basically everyone, with only a few exceptions within his team of thugs who move the product. This guy has all the money, and his bankroll just grows and grows. We are all here to contribute to his never-ending stash of cash.

Scoring our shit is done, now it's time to get out of here. The way out of the building is a bit creepier now that we are holding some serious stuff, and everyone here knows it. The junkies beg us as we walk by, grabbing at are ankles and clearly strung out beyond any rational thought. Luckily none of them are in any shape to actually attempt using physical force to rob us of our dope. We make it out fine; having a strong mind and keeping our eyes forward get us back to my car safely. First thing I do when we get in the car is lock the doors. Neither Brad nor I have any kind of weapon on us or in the car, so an altercation would most likely end in us giving up whatever we had just to save ourselves. The locked doors of the car only marginally protect us, but it makes us feel better for some reason nonetheless.

Once we hit the highway a wave of relief washes over the inside of the car. A wave so palpable you can feel it. The intensity of the last hour has surpassed all talking for the most part. The two of us have only exchanged verbal information when absolutely necessary, staying focused on making precise and calculated movements. One mistake can bring on an onslaught of consequences, and ultimately lead to death in the worst case scenario. You always have to be thinking about the worst case scenario – in order to avoid it that is. Brad turns around and hits play on the boom box as I quickly light two smokes at the same time and hand him one. We are out. We are done. We are golden.

Between my most recent paycheck, and Brad's Social Security check, we have enough heroin for two weeks, and a stash of blow to generate some more cash. I still to this day do not understand why Brad gets such a check, but I do know that it includes some sort of loophole in the system, which he has exploited. Sneaky fucker. We spent some serious cash today, but really got hooked up in the process. As long as I can keep my current position at work, I should be able to do this for awhile and be all set. Keeping the position, however, is another story. I'm being pushed to my limits daily as to how much bullshit I can take, one of these days I know I'm going to end up simply walking right off of the job. I'll deal with those consequences when they present themselves. For now it's time to focus on getting high.

The whole way home I am extremely conscience of anything that would bring attention to us from the local authorities. Always checking my speed to ensure that I'm not going too fast, or too slow for that matter. Using my turn signals at all times, and obeying traffic signs and lights perfectly. I don't want to give the police any reason at all to start sticking their snout in the car and making up some excuse to toss it. Our main goal is getting home safely so that we can enjoy our neat little scorpion stamped packet. I have the next two nights off, so recovery should be a piece of cake. Our last few nightly adventures have gone off without any trouble at all, and have been completely incredible. I find myself being able to actually control the urges in-between doses quite well now, knowing that I am going to be able to return in a short period of time. I have even been able to function when needed while high - to an extent. I wouldn't recommend dosing up and driving around town in the middle of an ice storm or anything, but I can deal with people on some level, and act normal enough to be convincing.

We pull up to the house and nobody seems to be home as there are no other cars in the driveway. This just makes things even easier. Today has been stellar on all fronts – I haven't felt happiness like this in quite some time. Brad told me this morning that he has a few girls that are going to come over tonight and hang out. One of them has a thing going with Brad at the moment, and she's bringing some of her friends. I don't usually get very excited about things like this, simply because meeting new people always seems to disappoint – girls especially. I have only met a few girls in my travels that have actually peaked my interest. The girlfriends that I have had in the past have helped me to understand the kind of person that I am, and the kind of person I am looking for ultimately. Transparency is not a personality trait that I seek, and tonight that's all I am expecting from our visitors. It will still be a fun night, just not with any relationship possibilities I'm sure.

Brad and I get inside and start getting ready to have our first fix. I lay everything necessary out on the coffee table and flip on the TV for some irrelevant background imagery to zone out to. Brad seems a bit anxious to shoot; I'll be supportive and not give him too much shit in the process. It's only a little bit after noon when I spike my vein for the first time – we managed to get a lot done today already. I'm proud of us both. We have every right to enjoy the next 18 hours to their fullest extent. And that is precisely what I intend to do.

16. Pain

I know that it is only Saturday night, but the delirium has me believing otherwise at times. The reminder that it is still only Saturday night is an excruciating thought that actually makes my head throb in response. That means I have over 24 hours of torment to go through. I can't take this. I find myself under the metal bed pushing against the wall with the palms of my hands. My clothes are torn and shredded from the constant rolling around on the floor. The injuries that I sustained from the attack have become completely irrelevant and replaced by the consuming pain from the withdrawal. Wet spots litter the floor where I have essentially thrown up nothing but spit and bile deep within my stomach. A tray full of piled up bread and spoiled meat sits in the corner from the three meals that have been slid through my door to me today. I want to crawl through the wall. I want to flush myself down the wretched toilet and swim out of a sewage drain 50 miles away from here. I want to disappear.

My muscles feel like floppy rubber bands that have lost all of their elasticity leaving me flailing about on the cold concrete floor. I can't feel anything on the outside, but everything inside is unbearable. My organs need to be replaced. My veins need to be flushed of their tainted blood supply and replaced with something useful. All of my body parts need to be replaced with mechanical equivalents that can actually withstand the pain that is traveling through them. I have become nothing.

The man down the hall may have been released. He may have been killed. He may have turned into a fixture in the hallway for all I know. I don't hear him anymore, but I can't tell if that is part of the illusion as well. Nothing seems real, and I doubt that anything actually is. My mind keeps telling me that I have been here since yesterday morning, but it literally feels like months. It feels like I have been put here deliberately to suffer. I don't even remember what I did that got me here; I stare at the underside of the bed and think for an eternity, still coming up with nothing. Something must be very wrong. I need help, from whoever will offer it. I need something from somebody, and yet nobody is there. Nobody is offering anything. This goes on forever.

I feel another attack from within coming on as the burn travels up my throat and spews onto the wall near my hands. Wrenching forward from the force I feel the crude concrete underneath me tear more skin from my exposed areas. I can't sleep. I can't eat. I can't do anything. I am stuck in a whirlpool of pain that has no end, beginning, or middle for that matter. It's a whirlpool of nothing that continues on within another whirlpool of nothing. My head spins and stops, spins and stops, spins and stops. I let go of the wall for a change and curl into an even tighter ball. I desperately want to roll over but I don't have the energy to do so. I might be able to work myself up to this movement if enough time passes, but right now it's completely out of the question. Here I will stay for now, a mass of blood, sweat and puke.

The sad thing about all of this is that it's only going to get worse. This constant pain will carry on and intensify as the hours pass, which will slow down in my head and feel like centuries. This illusion of time only makes the pain all that much worse to deal with, and all that much worse to anticipate. I have to stop thinking about it. I have to stop thinking altogether. If only I could stop the thoughts. If only I could better control my brain. What a powerful organ. I have already been using all of my energy to make sure that I don't think about anything too upsetting or personal. Desperately keeping my mind from wandering off with thoughts of my family or Nikki. I cannot accomplish anything while in this place, so there is no reason to harp on the things that will just make my pain worse or impossible to deal with. Not that I'm doing that good of a job right now. It takes a lot to stay away from these thoughts, especially when everything is my fault. Everything that has happened, and everything that has been ruined is entirely my fault. My way of life has ruined myself, and many others who care about me. I know this, even though they think I don't.

I start crawling to the center of the cell feeling like I am being crushed by the metal bed, which I have been underneath for hours. A sudden claustrophobic feeling took over and gave me a rush of adrenaline that allowed me to move a few feet away. I had to get away from the bed. The toilet is also making me nervous but I don't really have a reason why. I think it is due to the water inside, but I can't be certain. I can't be certain about anything at all. In the middle of the cell everything has changed. The ceiling feels like it is falling and within in millimeters of crushing me. More delirium. This is going to continue to haunt me throughout the weekend. Things that I know aren't real, but feel more real than the skin on my face. Doubting these things seems unnatural, even though I know better. It's the weirdest feeling to describe.

Another wave of sweat takes me over and I collapse with stomach pain. How can I still be throwing up? The burn takes form and travels up my esophagus once again. Without even having a reactive movement I wretch all over the floor to my side and set my head back down on the floor. I decide to take off the rag of a shirt that is still clutching to my shoulders in a desperate attempt to stay on. I'm hot and need to feel the cool floor against my skin for relief. Perhaps it will fend off the next attack of vomit. Let's hope.

I suddenly notice that my head feels like a balloon. Like it doesn't even fit in the room. A horrible pain pulses at my temples and makes me want to scream if it wouldn't hurt to do so. I open my mouth in response but nothing comes out, it can't.

Pain

I feel like at any moment my entire head is going to explode and paint the room with everything inside. Like the pressure has built to an amount that could take the whole building down if it was released. Honestly there is nothing more I'd love to do in this moment. Focus, focus, focus. This is starting to sound like a complete impossibility. But having made it almost halfway through this, I have to keep my eyes on getting out of here alive.

Staring at the blurry image of the ceiling I try to meditate once again. This time the fields that I envision are grayed in color and any vegetation is completely engulfed in flames. No life could sustain here. The giant rock wall is crumbling to pebbles and turns to dust before my eyes. The music is over due to piles of instruments that have been destroyed far beyond repair. A tear wells up and falls from my bloodshot eye. I am never going to get out of here alive.

17. Living

Having sex while high makes me feel nothing less than godly. Having built up a tolerance and more control I find myself able to remember just about everything from each session. The physical intensity of the act itself is magnified by a thousand, or so it seems. I must honestly say I have no desire to engage in an actual relationship at this point in my life. The last girl I was with left me with some serious scars. I don't feel like giving that much of myself to someone again only to have it all thrown right back at me with nothing more than a moment's notice. I have better things to focus my energies on right now anyways. Last night was fun though, it's good to feel that physical connection with someone every once in awhile.

I am rather enjoying the fact that I can remember things more clearly now while high. It makes each experience very fulfilling, both during and after. Everything shines so bright, I'm sad that I was not able to fully remember everything in the beginning. I have plenty of time to make up for that now though. A few stragglers have joined our group, from time to time stopping in to have a taste of our prized possession. Most of the people around here have never had anything that can even compare to the purity of dope like the scorpion. They come in and plop down cash without even thinking about it just to get some of our stash. Neither of us expected this at all, and now we have even one more way to make some extra money. If things keep going like this I'm going to have to make a weekly trip to the city to grab more shit. That sounds like a wonderful plan to me.

My car is starting to fall apart and has some issues that need to be addressed. Otherwise I am going to end up stranded somewhere, and most likely stranded somewhere very bad. It's time to address the most important issues and move on from there. I know a guy at a local shop that will tell me exactly what is critical to fix. I'm going to get ready and take that trip this morning, get it out of the way. With the extra cash that is coming in I'm sure that I can easily manage to get some things tuned up without a problem.

Putting on clothes has become quite different. I find myself looking for shirts that will completely cover up my arms so as to hide needle marks. Not something that I ever took into consideration in the past. After getting ready I run downstairs and call the shop to make sure that my friend is there. He tells me to bring it right over and they'll check it all out. Perfect. I hop in my hunk of junk and I'm off. Music blaring from the back seat, I have no worries in the world this morning. Last night was great and tonight will be too I'm sure. I'm actually being somewhat responsible right now, even if it is to ensure proper delivery of hard drugs. At least I have motivation.

I pull up to the garage and immediately have an epiphany. I bet that I could get some business from the workers here; perhaps I'll bring it up to my guy. I toss him my keys and he tells me to give him a call in about two hours. I'm off on foot, and not very far away from the house, but I think I might just walk around for a bit and take the really long way back. Get in touch with my city a little bit; it's been awhile since I've really walked around this place. I used to all of the time, back when I had no vehicle; you have to get around somehow.

Walking around these familiar streets I notice that I am viewing things from a different perspective. Having found a more meaningful purpose in my life now, the concepts that I once had in my head have seemed to disappear. I feel like a newborn seeing the world for the first time and through untainted eyes. I feel like a sponge ready to acquire all the knowledge that I can soak up. Even things as trivial as the storefronts that I have stared at for years seem completely different now. The smells are also suddenly unique. I stop for a moment and take everything in as deeply as I can. I seem to be walking with no real destination in mind, even though I am eventually going to end up back at the house. There are many ways to get there from here so I can walk up and down the side streets for as long as I want without actually getting off course. I have two hours before I need access to a phone, so I really don't care when I arrive. I am enjoying my leisurely walk through the city today far more than I ever have in the past.

For the first time in awhile – I feel good about myself. I feel good about this transition and have hope that it can actually work. I feel empowered and ready to start actually doing something constructive with my life. I'm ready to start getting myself on track with a real career and stop fucking around at the local grocery store making shit money, and essentially accomplishing nothing at all. I just hope that this time I can actually do it. This time I can actually stay on course and not get discouraged by the bullshit along the way. This time I can do it.

Making my way up toward Main Street I decide to duck into a small cafe and grab a coffee. I actually have some cash in my pocket, which is a first. I figured I might as well enjoy it and treat myself to something. Sometimes it's the smallest things in the world that can give such intense feelings of joy, even if it's only for a few moments. I feel very grounded right now, and really wish that everyday could be like this one. There is no anxiety floating around in my head. No longing to belong to something that I am not. No cares about what people think. I am simply being myself and walking around feeling a large sense of freedom.

I get back to the house and find Brad slumped over on the couch staring at the television. He's not watching anything in particular, but instead seems to be zoned out entirely not even noticing my entrance. The coffee table explains his current state, littered with all of the necessary tools for a fix. My guess is that he had about an hour, between waking up and getting high again, where he was actually sober. That's not good. Perhaps I should have a conversation with him later. We need to be watching out for each other at all costs when it comes to shit like this. The seriousness of what we are doing cannot be lost or else everything is going to come crashing down with a vengeance. Thinking about Brad definitely has put a bit of a damper on my mood.

I call the shop because it has been almost two hours. My guy tells me that I need new brakes, tie-rod ends, ball joints, and two front tires. He tells me that it'll be all done in the next two hours if I want, and that he can do it for 200 hundred bucks. I'm psyched to hear this and tell him to nail it. He has completely hooked me up with parts at cost and barely anything on the labor. There's a stack of cash sitting on the coffee table that Brad and I are treating as communal. Without my vehicle in tip-top shape, we have no way to score, so I quickly swipe what I need and pocket it. Brad doesn't even notice. He still doesn't even acknowledge my presence in the room. You would swear that he was sleeping, but his eyes are wide open, blinking on occasion. He took too much. Not too much to really cause any immediate harm, but too much to function. He must have been looking for a substantial escape this morning.

I decide to clean up the room a bit and keep an eye on Brad. I have to leave in little bit to make my way back to the shop and pick up my car. This makes me a little nervous. I really don't want to leave Brad unattended, but hopefully he'll be a bit more responsive before I leave. At least if I pick things up he won't have immediate access to more dope. This is obviously something that I need to pay more attention to. For some reason I didn't anticipate that he would already be high when I got back from the shop this morning. But now I know.

After I have successfully cleaned up anything incriminating, I realize that it's time to hit the road once again. I'm planning on taking another long walk to the shop just to enjoy the outdoors as much as I can. Brad has slumped even more to his side now and is completely out leaning over the arm of the couch. He's fine, just completely unconscious. I make the executive decision that he'll be ok until I get back, and set out into the street once again.

18. Impossible

Three men lift me up and try to stand me on my feet. My legs are incapable of bearing any weight. The life within me has been all but drained. I'm still alive because I can still feel pain, but I have no energy whatsoever to react to it. I am basically carried to a shower stall that luckily has a bench like seat lining all three walls. Stripped of my clothing, and sprayed with a powder like substance that I assume is soap, the water is turned on. At first I am overwhelmed with surprise as the feel of the water is completely foreign to me. Then it starts to feel good, but all I can do is sit there. The water that is spiraling toward the drain is a murky mixture of brown and red. The cuts on my head and on various parts of my body sting from the crude soap that has worked its way inside. I am assuming that it is early Monday morning. I am assuming that they are preparing me for my court appearance today. I am assuming that this is all real and that the weekend has passed.

"Monday?" I manage to utter to a guard.

"Its Sunday morning kid, man you're fucked up."

I was assuming wrong.

Almost as quickly as it happened I am being thrown back into my cell with some lost and found clothing tossed in after me. I am left in a pile on the floor where they set me down shivering from the cold concrete, being wet doesn't help much either. A towel seems to have been placed on my bed surprisingly, however it seems entirely too far away to retrieve. I feel as though the wind has been completely knocked out of me. Not knocked out of me, sucked out of me with not even a hidden pocket of air to spare. The terror that hit me once the guard responded is just starting to fully sink in. It's Sunday morning? How? I have been here forever. I have suffered an eternity. I have died a hundred times since I first walked into this room. I am about to die a thousand more.

There is nothing left to help me through this. I have exhausted every single option throughout the last day and a half; I have nothing left at all. Drained and whittled away to a mere outline of myself, I have no fight left. No desire to fight, and no desire for anything. I have puked all over this cell until the only thing left to throw up was sound itself. Hacking and wrenching my guts until the faint taste of blood makes its way into my mouth. My body has been left bruised and tattered from crawling across the hardened floor and grasping at whatever I can to stabilize myself. There is never enough there to help, and there never ever will be.

I have to shut off my brain. I have to stop thinking about anything and everything. I need to be put into a coma until all of this torment surpasses. But that's not going to happen. Suffer, suffer, suffer. That's all I can do. That's all I will do. 24 hours left and I will be out of this place, but still miles away from relief. The withdrawal will still have a hold on me; I can only hope that it will be slightly lessened. I can only hope that I will somehow be able to function or stand on my own. I can only hope that this pain and suffering will collapse even the tiniest bit. A single ounce of relief right now would make me happier than anyone on this planet. A single ounce of relief would probably enable me to stand up and actually walk around. I lie here and hope – what a crock of shit.

The remaining water has dried up on my body making me feel itchy and uncomfortable. I didn't think that I could possible feel any more uncomfortable than I already did – but I do. I attempt crawling to the pile of clothes that were left for me, but I find myself not getting anywhere at all. Getting colder by the second I curl up into a ball slowly and try willing myself into unconsciousness. Unsuccessful for what seems like weeks I somehow end up feeling even more drained than I did before.

Impossible

My grip on reality has slipped beyond repair as I am consumed by an image of myself chained to a wall with flaming torches all around me, and knives being slowly thrust into every exposed body part. I focus on the flame itself and drift into a never-ending hole of blackness.

19. Running

The following few weeks are filled with massive amounts of drug use and many trips to my new favorite city a mere 40 miles away. Picking up coke and peddling it back home has also really helped pad the income that Brad and I freely use for purchasing our luscious heroin. Everything has been going great with the exception of one fatal thing – Brad's heroin use. Brad's addiction has started to become a problem. We have actually had a few arguments regarding his carelessness while under the influence. His incessant use has also set us back a few times, with both money and product respectively. I try to keep things planned out pretty well so as to not actually run out of shit before making the trip out of town. Brad however has gone against our plans on numerous occasions and forced us to make tension filled trips to score out of sheer desperation and panic. We are on one of those trips right now.

I pull up to the familiar abandoned building and park in the first open spot that I see. All looks well on the outside, just like the last time we visited. Surprisingly I rarely notice law enforcement on this side of town. It seems as though they avoid it. As if they only come here when it's absolutely necessary, and not actively patrolling the streets. If Brad and I know about his place, the cops must know about it. I would assume that it is only a matter of time before it gets raided and is forced to shut its doors. For now, however, it seems like business as usual.

Brad makes the usual moves with the man behind the little cutout. Once again our inventory is replenished, I feel an immediate wave of relief - like a truck sized weight has been lifted off of my chest. All we have to do is make it back home.

Back in the car I suggest stopping for some food, a sudden surge of hunger roars through my stomach, and I can't actually remember the last time that I ate. Brad agrees halfheartedly and

Running

I pull into a local diner not far from the highway on-ramp. I've been to this particular diner before and always found their food to be cheap and extremely satisfying. It has been years since I've eaten here, so I am actually a little excited to see if anything has changed – my hopes are that it hasn't. I was right, even the booths themselves were still covered in the same red sparkly vinyl that is cracking due to their constant use. The cups, plates, napkins, and place mats – all still exactly the same. I find comfort in this. I'm glad that we stopped here.

Brad is flipping through the menu barely looking at it. I can tell that he is anxious to get home. He is anxious to use. Our last fix was last night. I came home from work and Brad already had everything out to cook up. I thought nothing of it, but found out why he was so assertive when I woke up this morning and discovered that we were completely out. Apparently he had been sneaking hits throughout the week when I wasn't around and had therefore, once again, deviated from the plan – causing this unexpected trip to cop. Luckily I had cash already stashed and ready to go. I learned early on to keep my hands on the money at all times rationing out only when I saw fit. Brad was a magician when it came to money, causing it to disappear with no explanation whatsoever.

I try to focus on the menu and not feed into Brad's insatiable urge to go home and shoot. The waitress promptly swings by with coffees for both of us and takes our orders. Brad mumbles something about sausage, which apparently she heard and wrote down with no questions at all, while I order pancakes and a poached egg. Finally it's time to relax for a few minutes while we wait. Brad immediately stands up and announces that he is going to the bathroom. I wave my hand and pick up the perfect cup of coffee that smells irresistible. It's been a long time since I have had some really good diner coffee, and at this moment I am completely content.

I start thinking about going to work tonight, contemplating calling out sick – I haven't done that in a few weeks. I feel like I should treat myself to an unexpected night off. Out of everything in my life right now, I despise work the most. I try so hard to just stick it out and think of other things while I am there in order to keep my mind occupied, but still the hours before I'm expected to be there fill me with dread. For me – there's nothing more depressing. I am fairly certain that I will be calling out sick tonight; the coffee is delicious and has helped me come to this decision.

Just then I notice Brad walking out of the bathroom with a strange smile on his face. My mind immediately starts racing trying to deduce what has caused his new found happiness. He sits back down across from me and I know in an instant. He's high.

"What the fuck?" I whisper to him sternly, not actually interested in an answer.

He doesn't answer, just continues to smile that stupid grin. His eyes are glazed over and he is using all of his energy to keep his head atop his shoulders. This is just wonderful. I had no idea that I would be spending the rest of this trip babysitting. I should have made sure that he left the shit in the car or that I had it – and where did he get a fucking needle? He must have had one. Fuck.

The waitress comes back with our food, which is another thing that I love about diners – their prompt service. I had forgotten all about our food though. This entire experience had just been completely ruined for me in an instant. As soon as he walked out of that bathroom – it was over. I can't believe that he actually went in there and shot up completely against all of the rules that we have put in place for very important reasons. His carelessness is going to really fuck things up for both of us, and I fear that it will be sooner rather than later.

I shake my head and start eating my food quickly, trying to not look suspicious while focusing on getting the fuck out of here as soon as possible. Brad fingers his sausage back and forth on his plate until I finally get his attention to stop. He decides that it will be better to just sit there and stare instead. I can't win. The bill comes and I plop down some cash eager to make our way out of the diner. It feels like everyone in the place is staring at the two of us, knowing exactly what is going on. It's then that I see the police cars pulling into the parking lot with their lights on.

When you are backed into a corner, it's amazing the decision making process that occurs. Electrodes fire off in your brain in rapid succession causing you to move without actually thinking about anything. A purely instinctual set of movements carefully planned in mere nanoseconds help to get you toward safer ground. I grab Brad from across the booth and drag him toward the rear exit with a profound sense of urgency. Luckily nobody was expecting our prompt reaction and had no time to even attempt stopping us.

"Did you leave something in the fucking bathroom?" I scream at him while we are running across the back parking lot. Brad tries to pick up his head and run as best as he can while I drag him by his hoodie.

"I think....I think... I left the needle...by mistake."

"Great! Just fucking great! We have to get out of sight – NOW!"

Running as fast as I can without losing my grip on Brad we manage to duck down an alleyway between two brick apartment buildings. I grab his hoodie, and my own, and rip them off tossing them behind a dumpster and continue on through the alley. We are still going to be very easy to spot and identify, but perhaps that will hinder things a little. The fact that Brad is high is making this much more difficult, he could be the reason why we end up getting pinched, then again if we do get pinched – he is the reason anyway. I'll worry about that later though – right now we have to find a way to disappear.

So far, since we left the diner, there has been no sign of police in any direction. We might have gotten lucky enough with our exit to actually pull this off. We hop the fence at the edge of the apartment complex, which sucked with Brad being completely uncoordinated, and cross the street just in time to catch a bus that was closing its doors at a bus stop. I walk up the stairs calmly handing the bus driver money for both of us as he looks at Brad and shoots me a glare.

"He's sick. I just have to get him home."

The doors close behind us with still no sign of the police. I drag Brad toward the back of the bus and push him into a seat near the window deliberately keeping him away from the general public that is also riding the bus. I surely hope that by some small miracle, nobody has made the connection between the two of us and my car that is still in the diner parking lot.

20. Sentence

The weekend is over. It must be. I find myself in the back of a police car once again, shackled at the wrists and ankles. I presume that we are on our way to the courthouse. Dressed in more hand me down clothes from the police station, I feel useless and permanently restrained. There's no sense in fighting anything at this point, I'll just take whatever comes and be happy, and hopefully that includes not going back to that dreaded concrete floor. I will surely die if that happens to be the case. I'll die right there in the courthouse in front of everyone. I'll die gladly.

Walking is a chore; I feel like I'm 170 years old and should have one of those four legged orthopedic walkers in front of me. The police officers are not amused at my snail like pace. Fuck them – they didn't help matters. If I had any saliva left in my mouth I'd spit on their fucking shoes on the way in – self important cocksuckers. Not a one of them could last 30 seconds in my shoes, before, after or during the arrest and containment. I have no respect for them, and the feeling is definitely mutual.

People like me are brought in through the rear of the court and ushered to a special area off to the side of the judge where you sit and wait for your case to be presented. This of course takes a long time, as they do these cases last. I am sitting there with my police entourage on either side of me waiting the excruciating three hours of bullshit before I am finally told to stand. The judge looks at me and makes his own conclusions within seconds. This is why the justice system is completely fucked and totally biased. Another wave of hopelessness and sheer anger washes over me. It's all I can do to keep from screaming and bursting into a full blown tantrum. I know that will land me right back in that cell again – and I am not going to do anything that will help facilitate that.

The judge refers to me as a menace, and a slight on society. His words. I get nailed with a 1200 dollar fine for an unrelated charge that occurred a few months ago, however I never showed up for the court date. I also get two years probation that will include monthly piss tests and meeting with a PO every few weeks. Finally I am court ordered to a rehabilitation facility effective immediately for two weeks. Here we go again. The only relief in that punishment is the meds that I'll get to help curve the withdrawal. Other than that rehab is a total fucking drag. Surrounded by people who either have no desire to get clean, or have suddenly found Jesus. There is nothing more annoying than a newly religious person, especially if they used to be a junkie. They just replace their substance addiction with this new, just as unhealthy one. I'd rather be physically addicted to something than brainwashed any day of the week. Heroin might put me in danger on a regular basis, but I still have my mind. Not having it scares me more than anything else on this planet.

I am walked back out to cruiser and once again stuffed into the tiny backseat. This time without the shackles – apparently I am magically no longer a threat – because the judge said so. If they only knew the thoughts that were actually going through my head. If they only knew how badly I would love to hurt either one of these police officers right now, just to knock them off of their high horse. The arrogance exuding off of them stinks, and makes my eyes water like staring at a rotten onion. Stay calm. In a few minutes I won't have to be in their presence anymore. I will however have to sit and listen to the philosophies of some earthy crunchy counselor who thinks that they know every single facet of my life because they were once an addict as well. Whatever. Give me some meds and a bed, and leave me alone. That's all the rehab I need.

We pull up and once again the bastards in blue reluctantly help me hobble to the front lobby where two humanitarian types take over the task. The irony of the four of them standing there is blaring. Two people whose main goal is to make life miserable for as many as they can, and two who try to accomplish the exact opposite. All of them are wrong and too much to take, if someone could show up somewhere right in the middle, it would be perfect. That's obviously way too much to ask for. The cops explain that I am not allowed to leave – and finally they do. A gigantic sense of freedom takes over me as I sit in an overstuffed chair not wanting to ever move again. I just want to feel this padded fabric against my body for all of eternity. The difference between this chair and all of the places that I have been since Friday morning is exponential. I could melt right here and I'd forever be happy.

The two ladies that are about to help me to my new room are aware of my sudden comfort and decide to sit down across from me in order to process a little bit of the immediate paperwork. Trivial things like my name and address, which is easy because I don't live anywhere, are asked of me slowly and patiently. This is such a change. So much so I almost feel like crying. I have arrived in a place that very closely resembles my idea of heaven at the moment. After that is done and out of the way there seems to be a sense of urgency for me to consume some meds. I certainly have no issues with this, as I am ready for any kind of relief that can be administered to me at this time. The cuts and scrapes about my body are starting to hurt more and more as the feeling in my limbs slowly fades back in. The detox period is starting to wear off. Most of my physical dependency to heroin has left my system. The mental craving however is there in full force. I have to fight it with every step that I take and every thought that I have. The meds will help with this a lot, and I can't wait to get them.

Once I down my meds it's time for some much needed rest, and in a comfortable environment. Having already gone through the drastic effects of the withdrawal I should have an easier time getting some sleep. I have a lot to deal with once I wake up. Nikki still has no idea where I am even if she did find out that I was picked up, because now I will be here for two weeks. I have to find a way to contact someone that can relay the message to her so that she isn't worried sick. That's assuming that everything is going well on her end and she hasn't gotten picked up herself. Similar situations have happened in the past - landing a few nights in jail is pretty much inevitable. Especially when the two of us get broken up, out here you need as much support as you can get from whomever you can get it from, losing a piece of that support can drastically change things for the worse.

  I'm going to have to bite the bullet and call a family member. I hate doing this because of what I am putting everyone through. My Mom is a wreck all of the time, especially when I talk to her on the phone. She worries all of the time, and I don't blame her. If she was privy to half of what goes on day to day in my life I'm sure she'd never even sleep. The best way to do this will be to call my brother. He'll get the people who need to know informed, and if need be come down here. That's what I am going to do in the morning; luckily the cops were nice enough to leave me here with my little manila envelope, which has all of my important phone numbers in it.

  I can feel the meds soothing my brain, this feeling is also very foreign to me and I doubt I have ever felt anything quite as exquisite. I imagine a million swords that at one time pierced my skin and cut into my organs all being pulled out at once with the wounds closing up behind them. Relief like no other cradles me. As much as I don't want to be here, it's the best place for me at the moment. This bed feels like a water bed compared to what I am used to, I haven't even touched one in over two months. It's miraculous how low you can allow yourself to get, and what little you can survive on if need be. We don't push our minds or bodies nearly as far as we are capable of.

21. Cinema

nce we have gotten a few miles away, and are near the shopping hub of the city, I decide it's time to disembark. I haul Brad to his feet, who has been sleeping for the last five minutes, and all but carry him down the walkway and off of the bus, catching another accusatory glare from the asshole bus driver. It's impossible to do anything around here. I have decided that we need to hang out here until it starts to get dark out and then sneak back to the diner to see if my car is gone. I really have a mess on my hands now.

Mixing in with the crowd sounds a lot easier than it actually is. This is not a crowd that Brad and I can mix in with visually, even if he wasn't ripped out of his mind. In this crowd we are seen as thieves. Parents pull their children closer to them as we approach. Store owners lock their eyes on us even when we are just near the entrances. This is supposed to be the best place for us to be, but it's not. In a lot of ways it's worse than where we came from, now having millions of suspicious eyes piecing together judgmental thoughts in their heads. Where do you go when there is no place left to hide? You go to the movies.

Standing in line at the theater anxiously waiting to buy tickets, I quickly pick a movie that is starting soon. At malls like this the theaters are usually of substantial size with multiple times hitting almost every hour. The more popular movies have multiple theaters as well, which means less people throughout, especially if they have already opened a week or so ago. I choose one of those. Pretending that Brad is my slightly retarded family member I purchase two tickets and grab a couple of sodas at the concession stand to appear normal. Off to the theater we go. This will be the most perfect hiding spot for the next two and a half hours, and by that time we will be approaching nightfall. Free and clear to go back outside once again.

Brad will at least be able to get some sleep in here, and perhaps come out of his robot-like state by the time the movie is over. I need him to be in better shape for so many reasons. First of all he is completely blowing our cover with every step we make. The public doesn't do well with someone acting the way he has been. Even if that was actually how he was at all times. It definitely draws far too much attention, which is the very last thing we need at this time. Trying to lay low with the uncoordinated Siamese twin is next to impossible. He better snap out of it, or I'm going to shove coke up his nose until his heart is visibly pounding out of his chest. Fucker.

The movie finally comes on, but I am actually glad that it took so long, that means that we are going to be in here for awhile, and that's a good thing. The longer the better, if it was up to me we'd be in here for five hours, but we can't be so I'll take what I can get. The lights have gone completely out and the movie is rolling. I finally feel safe for the first time since we ran out of the diner. I lean my head back against the seat and close my eyes. Being able to think clearly for the first time in hours I start to become nervous about my previous plan of looking for the car. I have come to the conclusion that we need to drive by it rather than be on foot. I have to call someone to come down here and help us out. Who should I call? Who can I get away with not telling all of the details to? And if the car is gone, how the fuck am I going to get it back? This sucks. There is a girl back home that I know quite well who knows not to ask too many questions. She's not a fan of Brad, but I think since it's me I can get her to hook me up this one time, especially if I tell him that he has to keep his mouth shut, it is his fault after all that we are even in this mess. I'll call her after the movie.

Aside from Brad and I there are six other people in the theater, it really couldn't have worked out much better than this. I'm very thankful that the idea even came to me when it did, otherwise who knows how much longer we would have made it out in the endless sea of people. Complacent is the only way to go through life without attracting attention. How you look and how you act sets off alarms in these people's heads that immediately shouts "danger". Ironically I'm no more a danger to anyone in this building than the shitty food they are all stuffing their faces with in between feeding their own addiction of buying useless shit. It's all about what is and isn't acceptable, perhaps in a thousand years it will all flip flop and be different. Not that that matters right now, it's not something I'll ever witness with my own two eyes, even if I do manage to live until I'm 82.

Still thinking about how I am going to convince my friend Kristen to make the trek out here, I find myself drifting in and out of consciousness. It's been a long day and I have a feeling that it's going to be a long night as well, depending on what ends up happening. I'm not going to fight to stay awake as I may need all of the energy I can get. Sleeping also helps to pass the time faster as I am completely uninterested in the actual movie itself. Luckily Brad has been lightly snoring away since the minute we sat down, I'm convinced he has no idea that we are even at the movies - he probably thinks we're still home.

I wake up to the sound of music and realize that the credits are rolling on the screen. It's time to leave, and make some calls. I quickly walk Brad to a drug store within the mall to grab some smokes and get some change for the payphone outside. Three dollars worth of quarters should be sufficient. The first call I make is to Kristen, I need to convince her quickly so that she can start driving soon, so as to not take all night getting here. With a little persuasion and a promise to write a short two page essay on the issues with current musical trends for one of her college courses, she gladly gets in her car and hits the road. One task done. The next phone call is to work, I guess I had decided to call out sick tonight for a reason. Right now I certainly had one. They didn't seem too happy on the phone, but

I put on my best act even coughing when I told them my name forcing myself to give it a second time. The lady on the other end told me to feel better before she hung up the phone; obviously she believed enough of it. Besides, it's not like I work for 911 dispatch and 32 people might die tonight because I'm not at work. I'm sure they can find someone else to scan my usual load of groceries for the night, or not, either way it won't make a single difference to the world.

      Brad has finally started coming to his senses, and I start filling him in with the events of the day. At first his reaction is to start laughing uncontrollably, I then punch him in the arm he's always stuffing dope into, which hurts like a bastard. He stops laughing. Brad's disregard for wrong doing was fine with me, but not when I'm the one that is left picking up all of the slack so we don't get busted. I can't help but wonder if he'd do the same if the situation was reversed, or if he'd even be capable of it. This irritates me. I warn him that Kristen is coming to give us a ride by the diner to see if my car is still there, and that if he says a single word to her he's getting another punch, only this time harder. I tell him that I will continue to do so for every single word that follows as well, until his entire arm is black and blue and throbbing uncontrollably, and then I'll hit it again. I'm in no mood for his shit right now, and have no tolerance for it at all.

      Kristen pulls up glaring at Brad, and I jump in the front seat while he climbs in the back. We're only ten minutes from the diner, so this should go very quickly. I toss her a 20 dollar bill to cover her gas, which she refuses, but I insist stuffing it into her bra – we have that kind of relationship. As we approach the diner I notice that there are about five cars in the lot and mine is still there. I can't believe it; however I am still very leery to go near it. I toss Brad the keys and tell him that he's going to get it. We park down the street from the diner, and I set him out on foot to inconspicuously retrieve my car. Surprisingly, five minutes later, he pulls up behind Kristen and me without a problem whatsoever. He must have been able to get in and take off without anyone recognizing him, probably due to a shift change. The cops and workers at the diner must have assumed that we were on foot, therefore not making the connection to my car.

I lean over and peck Kristen on the cheek assuring her that I'll give her a call in a day or so to catch up with her on that paper she needs written. Thanking her profusely once again I step out of the car and walk over to mine.

"Get over in the passenger seat." I say in a demanding tone.

"I'm sick of riding man, I want to drive us home for once." Brad's whining voice replies.

"Like fucking hell!" I hold out my palm with the scorpion stamp staring him square in the face, his eyes widen ever so slightly. "You ever want to see this shit again...you'll move your ass over to that seat." It's tough love today out here under the stars. Brad climbs over the shifter clumsily as I slide in and drive toward the on-ramp.

22. Captivity

The morning has come, and I am starting to feel a lot better. That's usually how it goes in these places, but this time is different due to the events that occurred right beforehand. I needed this bad, and not really for the drug addiction itself, but for everything else that happened to me physically. A few more days in that cell and I would have been as good as dead - I'm convinced of that. I do need to stop using, but I know what always happens when I leave these places. The hold it has on me is too strong, I'll go right back to it as soon as I'm out. I'm not trying to be negative, just realistic. I have found that it's better to not have a false sense of hope – it only makes you fall that much harder. I suppose it's that age old expression of just not being ready to give it up on the inside. I'll just have to see what happens this time.

There are a few things about this arrangement that do indeed put dampers on things for me. First of all there are scheduled cigarette breaks. The one drug that they don't take away from the visitors here is nicotine. I think that would be considered cruel and unusual punishment. It would simply be too much to ask of someone with a serious addiction to kick smoking as well. It would never ever happen. The other thing that is hard to get is phone time. You are only given a few opportunities to use the phone and they are at timed intervals. This makes deciding who you are going to call, and for what purpose, a little difficult. Other than those two things the rest of it is pretty much a piece of cake. Having to attend meetings can be quite boring, but it's certainly not as painful as being in jail. Luckily I don't have a job to worry about. Not having to explain a two week hiatus this time will certainly make things easier. The first time this happened I lost my job, which was probably going to happen soon anyways.

Captivity

First things first – I have to call my brother. He'll deal with my Mom and the rest of my family, and try to get a message out to Nikki for me. He's not going to be happy to hear what went down, but at least he'll be happy that I'm back in rehab. He's always trying to get me to go, but at least he's not overly annoying about it like everyone else. Being more on my level, he sees things a bit more clearly than the rest. That's why I actually feel comfortable calling him right now and nobody else. The phone rings twice and he picks up. I explain what's going on and he asks me minimal details, which is nice. He has the means to ultimately get in touch with Nikki's parents and find out what's going on there. I'll give him another call tomorrow to check in on things; hopefully nothing too bad has happened.

Done with the phone it's time to take care of some paperwork that I wasn't able to get to yesterday when I got here. I'm not overly enthused by this, but I suppose it has to be done. I get back to my room and start filling things out. I've done this so many times before in the past. With only one time actually feeling like I was going to get somewhere. That was a few months ago, and boy was I ever wrong. I came out of rehab dying to use again, and that's exactly what I did. That was the time I was the most serious about staying clean, which is why I have never held out much hope for all of the other subsequent visits.

I notice that a nice yellow folder with built in pockets has been left in my room – filled with guidelines and regulations of the facility. All the same literature that I have seen a dozen times before, just with a different name and logo typed out on the top of each paper. I quickly scan through to note any subtle differences that might pertain to my schedule directly. There really aren't any except for slightly skewed time intervals. Just another routine to get used to over the next few days. Easy enough.

I need to go through an intake interview in an hour or so. This will most likely be one of the most painful things that I have to endure here. Not because it upsets me, but because I have to explain myself, yet again, to someone who already thinks that they have all of the answers. The solutions to my problems aren't going to jump out of a text book and suddenly make everything ok. You can counsel me all day long, but I still have to go back out there. I still have to go back out into the real world and deal with real life. Even though my choices have made a mess of things, they are also the choices that have helped keep me alive. I know that my addiction is a problem. I know that it has consumed my life more than anything ever has, and probably ever will. I know that every day I put my own life at risk in order to support it and feed it. This knowledge will not make it all just go away. Only I can do that. I need to develop a real plan that is logical and realistic before I can even begin to think about getting off of this shit. I've tried a lot of things in the past and still haven't quite gotten there. I haven't given up yet though, I'll leave here trying, and that's all that I can promise.

I walk into my assigned counselor's office right on time and take a seat in front of the desk. Two minutes later she enters. I'm so glad that it's a woman. They tend to take some sort of pity on me while I tell my story – men just act like closet homosexuals. This is much easier to deal with. I can win her over with a little bit of charm and make her realize that I'm a real person, with at least of half my brain, that isn't just running around causing a ruckus for the sheer fun of it. I tell this woman the cliff notes version of my sad tale, and she seems very interested. I focus on the failed attempts of staying clean and my current residence that has four wheels and a steering wheel. Every so often I glance at the clock on the wall, anxious to not miss the smoke break that begins at 12:40 and lasts for 15 minutes. The next one isn't until 2:40 so there's no way I'm going to let anything get in the way of nailing it. I start to wrap things up quickly, but not in a manner that could be mistaken as me being in a hurry. She buys everything hook, line, and sinker – immediately treating me as a human being rather than another zombie-like addict. I'm surprised at first, and then proud of myself.

After my smoke break I have an hour of group activity to suffer through. Then time allotted for written assignments before the next smoke break 40 minutes later. One more hour of group activity followed by another 30 minutes for written assignments. Then we have patient presentations – those are usually fun. 5:00pm brings dinner, or "supper" if you are reading the schedule, but something about that word makes me feel like I'm ten years old. 6:00pm, just when it seems like you haven't had a cigarette in a hundred years, there's another smoke break. That stretch from 3:00pm to 6:00pm is completely murderous, and almost always the worst time of the day. Incidentally it's also usually when someone melts down and goes nutty in front of the entire floor. This also helps to break up the monotony. Group activity shows up again, immediately following, from 6:30pm to 7:30pm. Another smoke break shows itself at 7:40pm, which is the second to last one for the evening. Group activity slides in once again at the 8:00pm slot leaving a 9:00pm break that doesn't include smoking for 15 minutes. 9:15pm is especially weird, being occupied by counselor facilitated meditation, which also lasts for 15 minutes, thankfully. 9:40pm is the last smoke break of the evening – barring special instructions, if granted, for the overnight hours. You have free time until 10:30pm to roam around and do what you wish, when at that time you are supposed to be in your room, reflecting apparently. Finally 11:00pm brings lights out, and that's pretty much it.

That will basically be how my next 13 days in here will go, with only slight variations from time to time. I'll probably pick up a few new friends along the way, but certainly not as many as

I used to, as I have gotten used to keeping to myself for the most part while in here. Friends in here are sometimes dangerous, sometimes good, but usually a bad idea. It takes a lot of work to really weed out the people you should definitely stay away from, and allow the ones that won't be detrimental to you progress to get just close enough without causing too many issues. It's a constant full time job and at times exhausting. Not worrying too much about that at the moment I put out my second smoke and get ready for my first group activity of the day. I walk into the large classroom like area and immediately recognize three people. This is going to be an interesting couple of weeks.

23. Force

It feels good to sleep tonight. After everything that went down earlier, I feel lucky to have gotten away with our little episode at the diner. I am still reeling at Brad's stupidity and complete disregard for his actions. He didn't mention it on the way home and still hasn't, but I know that deep down inside he finds it all somewhat amusing. Brad is drawn to everything that he shouldn't be doing. It excites him on some level, and then he's proud about it afterward – always telling stories at gatherings to get a rise out of everyone present. I always knew that he was this way, but for some reason I didn't really see this coming. I suppose that's my own fault – I should have seen it from 100 miles away. But I didn't. I need to find some way out of this, or at least come up with an alternative to the "Brad" way of life.

I put it all aside for the moment and decide to get some much needed rest – clean as a whistle having had plenty of excitement for one day. I'm glad that I have the self control to resist using, even if it is for just this one night. I stashed the remaining cash and all of the drugs in a secret undisclosed location in my room, and Brad didn't even mention getting high again. I know he didn't learn his lesson, but at least he's not pushing my buttons. With that being my last thought – I quietly drift off to sleep.

My dreams tonight are filled with endless arrays of colors that swirl and morph into elaborate geometric shapes like that of a kaleidoscope. For some reason this barrage of colors and shapes are extremely comforting and afford me some of the best sleep that I have gotten in years. I stare at the intricacies of their designs and follow their slow mutation into the next elaboration that they create. My mind is locked in awe and blank with all thought. Peacefulness exudes from this wondrous performance with every calculated movement that occurs in my mind. I have found another place that I never ever want to leave. To be frozen here forever would be a utopia like no other. If only that was a possibility.

I awake, disoriented at first, and realize that I am safely in my bed, and that it is still very early in the morning – 3:00am to be exact. I climb out of my bed and decide to use the bathroom as quickly as possible. Back in bed I find a new comfortable position and fall back asleep without hesitation. This time however, the dreams are different. I find myself walking through a tunnel with no doors or points of entry of any kind. Every few feet I am confronted by a different person who isn't actually there. An apparition of sorts used for each character that I come across. Their faces float toward me slowly and then increase in speed with each step that I take toward them. As they get within a few feet they start urgently speaking to me mumbling incomprehensible words that I cannot understand or make out. They each want something, but I can't figure out what. This goes on for quite some time. Finally I reach the end of the tunnel, exhausted and frustrated, only to find an enormous waste land of used needles. A sign is hanging on the tunnel wall above them which reads "Yours is in there". I stare down at the empty needles in terror, overcome with the need to find my needle and get a fix. The used needles that are strewn about are caked with dried blood and traces of my favorite drug that didn't quite make it all the way out. I start to carefully move the ones on top to the side of me, cautions to not get stuck by any of them. This has become my task until I come across the one needle that has my name on it. Finally after handling hundreds of used needles I reach the floor of the tunnel only to find another sign. This one reads "Just Kidding". I collapse in pain and anguish flailing about in all of the used needles on the floor – screaming and frantically swimming my way through them with my hands. Needles litter my body at random points and strings of blood start flowing from their entry points. Just when I can't take it any longer - I wake up.

Sweat has drenched everything around me – the sheets, the bed, and my boxers – everything. I am in a state of shock as I slowly realize that it was all just a dream. Anxiety starts to fade away slowly, leaving me feeling only mildly better. I lift up my sweat soaked hands and watch as they tremble uncontrollably. The clock says 3:52am. Damn. My stomach is turning and almost queasy. My head feels like it weighs 40 pounds, and takes much effort to hold up. I need a fix. And I need one soon. Fuck. I stumble over to the secret hiding place in my closet. Reaching under a mound of clothes I pull out a small wooden box that has a combination lock built into the front of it, lining up the numbers one by one frantically to read 5446. I'm in. The scorpion stamp is the first thing that I see, along with everything else necessary – syringe, lighter, metal cap. I open the packet and tap some dope out into the cap getting ready to cook. My hand is shaking so bad I almost can't get my shit cooked without spilling it all over the floor; this also fills me with anxiety, making the tremors even harder to control. I can't believe the ferocity behind it all. I need to focus, and spike my vein without missing - that would suck just as bad. Accidentally shooting in a muscle hurts like hell usually, and defeats the point. Staring at the bright blue line under the skin in the crook of my arm I slowly bring the needle closer and closer. Sweat pours off of my head and drips into my eyes. I have to put the needle down and clear my vision with a shirt that is on the floor near my bed. Let's try this again. Deep breath. I can feel the tiny prick and then my nerves start to calm. I take it all in one swift plunge, and lean back against the wall near the closet. The needle is still stuck in my arm, and I don't care. I don't care about anything actually as I stare at the ceiling and feel my body cure itself within seconds. My tremors stabilize, my stomach stops churning, and the sweating all but stops within an instant. I exhale deeply and feel a gigantic smile stretch across my face. I needed that.

Everything has returned to normal. The dream has disappeared from my memory, thankfully, that was horrible. The need to use was insurmountable. I was completely overcome and had no choice at all. I made no conscious decision to run to the closet and break into the secret hiding place. My body just reacted out of instinct. Like a dehydrated horse galloping to a pond. Like a dog that has been given 50 pounds of raw bloody steak and can't stop eating no matter how full he gets. All control had been sucked out of my body the moment I woke up from that nightmare. This might sound like a complaint, but in this very moment, it is anything but, as I float around the room feeling the beauty in all that is around me.

24. Boiling Point

The first few days of the rehab stint go off without too much weirdness. Things always get weird though – no matter what. The three people that I recognized from that first meeting have for the most part kept their distance. They aren't people that I'm down with, but we co-exist for the most part without any issues. I'd rather it be this way. Recognizing someone that you know, and actually get along with, tends to make things a bit difficult and awkward. There's a sense of defeat when you end up in a place like this, as well as profound feeling of shame that goes along with it. It's painful for people who actually know you to be there with you at the same time, going through their own strange version of substance abuse. In a lot of ways it makes things more difficult because you knew them already and have your own opinions of them in your head. That's just my perspective though, which could very easily be totally fucked. Who knows?

Today could have started better. The coffee in this place is starting to kill me, bordering on the edge of barely acceptable and absolute shit. Today it was absolute shit. I even waited for a fresh batch to be brewed and quickly found out that it was just as shitty. The same asshole must have made both. Damn. This puts me on edge right away and it's all I can do to wait for the next smoke break. I am going to smoke as much as I possibly can when it does finally arrive, hopefully inducing a nicotine coma. My luck would never allow such a thing however.

Today is going to be long. The longest one since I got here. I can feel it. The urge to find dope is rising with every minute as well. The meds helped immensely when I arrived because of the intense physical withdrawal and subsequent detoxification. Now however they are only helping to a certain extent with my mental craving for heroin. I keep trying to find other ways to get my mind off of it, even if it's for just while I am in here. Jonesing for a fix while in here is stupid, because I will never ever get one. Therefore it's a waste of my time and just makes things even harder, so instead I have been smoking my head off whenever I get a chance and trying to stay busy. The coffee actually helps as well, but not today, which really sucks. It's amazing how much the small things matter when you are trying to keep away from something as controlling as heroin. Every little bit helps, no matter how insignificant it may seem to someone else.

I'm outside sucking down nicotine like it's my job. Wanting to eat the filters when I am done just in case there is more to be had hiding inside the small fibers. I quickly light another one and hope that I have time for a third. My method is not that much different than anyone else who is out here in the freezing cold sucking down smokes. You would swear that the entire rehab unit migrates outside during every single smoke break. Sometimes there's actual congestion at the double doors that carrel us out to the designated courtyard. I find it to be somewhat amusing. All of us fiends, going outside to partake in our accepted addiction. It's very contradictory in so many ways. Either way, I'm very thankful that we have these breaks; I can't even fathom not smoking.

It's time to go sit through another group story. Today it's an alcoholic who ruined his life, as always. Lost his house, job, family, bla bla bla. It's just another scrambled version of every single story that gets told during AA meetings. I know that I should on some level, but I can't even begin to bring myself to care. Same old shit all the time. It doesn't help me at all; it just makes me more bored, which in turn makes my mind wander. Everything I look at reminds me of my drug. The pens look like needles. The packets of sugar remind me of dope. The spoons, and caps, and random pieces of metal. The rubber bands lying around on tables just itching to be wrapped around my biceps until the veins burst out of my forearms. The belts that have become so visible from the alcoholics who have so diligently tucked in their shirts - as if this somehow makes them a more respectable member or society - also have the same effect of me. Even the couches make me feel like I should be propped up against one on the floor of Dave's house with a needle hanging out of my arm. Everywhere I look I am reminded, and everywhere I turn I am told no. I am starting to lose it and need to get out of here. I can't be here any longer.

I start screaming right there in the middle of group activity. Tears streaming down my face and no understandable words coming out of my mouth – everybody stares in silence.

"Has this place really become this dead? Have you all just turned into corpses?" "Stop being so controlled by your fears!!!" "Let go and grow the fuck up, take control of something for once!!" I walk throughout the classroom pointing at random people. I feel like I have lost my mind. Either that, or I haven't, and everyone else has. No matter how you slice it – something is very, very wrong here, and it's only going to get worse. I grab the underside of the banquet table that has the shitty coffee on top and all of the cups and condiments next to it, and lift with all my force overturning the whole mess onto the floor. That's when I feel the arms around my shoulders and a needle entering my bicep. Not the needle I was looking for – but I'll take it. Fuckers.

I wake up in a room that has minimal light and a locked door. Good. As long as there are no legal repercussions to my little outburst, this is better. It's not like the cell at all, it's almost a real room just more confined and locked. I am visited by a staff member an hour or so after I wake up, who tells me that I will be here for the rest of the day and released in the morning. I will have to issue an apology to the entire floor, staff included, for disrupting group and harassing my fellow friends on the floor. This apology will have to be presented in front of everyone on the floor and is expected to be a well written speech of about

500 words or less. I will be given a few days to prepare – not that I need it. I feel like standing up in front of everyone and screaming "FUCK YOU" 250 times, but I have a feeling that I wouldn't get much applause for that. I'll just have to save that speech for another time.

For now I am supposed to sit here and reflect on what I did. Apparently this is punishment for some, not for me. I'm exactly where I want to be, away from the madness and alone at last with my own thoughts. I know exactly what I did – to an extent. I didn't expect the mental breakdown and the sudden crying, but I certainly loved turning over that fucking table and exposing everyone for exactly who they really are. So sick of the "normal" formulated way that has been accepted as a solution to these extremely complicated problems. These are people's lives that this place is screwing with. I really don't think that any of it is right at all. I feel as though I will be dead if I succumb to the propaganda. I will no longer be myself, and I will completely lose all free will - or the ability to think on my own for that matter. I will do whatever I can to ensure that this never happens to me, even if that means having to kick this habit completely on my own and without the help of places like these. I am not going to suddenly find my higher power and give my mind over to religion. I am not going to suddenly think that all of the thoughts I have had, and currently still have, are wrong and that I need to learn to think like somebody else. These notions scare me way more than any substance addiction that there is.

25. Bonds

When I finally come to my senses it's 7:30 in the morning. There's no sun to be seen in any direction, it's an overcast day outside, gray and damp. I like that. I peel myself off of the floor of my room and make my way downstairs. Brad is already up and itching for a fix as soon as he hears signs of life coming from my room. I'm surprised that he didn't knock my door down hours ago out of desperation. I already have the shit in my hand when I see him sitting on the couch tapping his fingers on the coffee table and staring at the staircase. I toss the packet to him and he smiles deeply with a sigh of relief. I walk into the kitchen looking for anything edible to quickly get into my stomach. A bag of chips from yesterday is sitting on the counter; I take them and walk back into the living room. Brad already has the needle in his arm. He's going to be no fun today at all.

I go back upstairs to take a shower and decide immediately that I'm going to try breaking my brother out of school today for a ride through the woods. I haven't seen or talked to him since the day I moved in a month ago. He helped me with what little boxes that I had, and we all hung out drinking listening to the newest Wu-Tang album before I brought him back home. I can't think of anyone else who I'd rather spend the day with today, and it's been a long time anyways. I'll hit his pager when I get out of the shower.

I have to actually go to work tonight which already bothers me, even though I have the entire day still until I actually have to show up there. I have no plans to use all day however, that way I can treat myself when I get home. I quickly get dressed and run downstairs to grab the dope from Brad so that I can stash it back in the little wooden box. He's already comatose staring at some terrible morning news show. Apparently that's the only way to get through that kind of television. Certainly understandable. I bring the shit back upstairs, and page my brother with the appropriate code to let him know that I'll pick him up at the school – we've done this before. With Dave and his fiance both at work during the day, Brad is basically left squatting at the house all alone, he always manages to get himself in a freeloading type situation. I'm starting to resent him a little bit.

Once I'm in the car I forget all about Brad and head out toward the high school I used to attend. By the time I get there my brother will be waiting for me in the far corner of the student parking lot. I still don't quite know how he pulls it off, but he manages to get out of school whenever he pleases and never gets in any kind of trouble at all. I used to just flat out skip and deal with the consequences later, which always sucked, but it was worth it every time. My brother on the other hand is much more conniving than I am, and always finds a way to cover his tracks so that there are no consequences to deal with. Of course every once in a while things don't go quite as planned, but that's expected, for the most part he ends up clean as a whistle. It's an admirable quality really.

I show up, and sure enough he's standing there already having a smoke. I don't even bother asking what strings he pulled this time as he jumps in the passenger seat. We are going to take a ride and grab some lunch a few towns over. I have a joint rolled and ready in the glove compartment, which my brother swiftly removes and lights up as we cruise through the wooded roads on the outskirts of town.

My brother and I have a lot in common, even though he's a few years younger than me. We share a lot of the same beliefs and ideals, and listen to basically the same kind of music, which is very important. He does not know about my heroin use, nobody does actually, except for Brad. He knows a lot, but not that. I'm not sure how he'd react to it, but I have a feeling that he wouldn't be too happy. Sometimes he acts like he's 45 years old or something, and I'm sure he'd try fathering me about it right away. That's definitely a conversation that can wait.

We chat it up a little bit about whatever interesting things have happened in the past couple of weeks, but soon we both just relax and enjoy the ride, listening to music on the way to yet another diner about 45 minutes away from the high school. The atmosphere in the car is perfect, and the mood of the day itself is fitting as well. Calm and quiet outside, I wish I could just do this for the rest of the week and never go back to anything real.

Arriving at the diner in what seems like record time; we get out of the car slowly and walk inside, both a little high and in no hurry whatsoever. The day is young still, and I am glad that this is what I decided to do this morning. Sometimes I forget how much I like spending time with him as opposed to most of my degenerate friends. I definitely have to make an effort to do this more often.

After drinking coffee by the gallon and downing a bunch of breakfast food, we decide to hit the road. We spent an hour and a half at the diner; my brother filled me in about things back home, and I told him some tales of Brad acting like a retard. He always gets a kick out of his stories, because Brad always does things exactly the way that he wouldn't – thankfully. I have never had to "watch out" for my little brother, I have no idea where he learned half of his tricks, and really wish that I could take credit for them, but I can't. If I didn't think it was weird I'd ask his thoughts on my current situation because I'm sure he'd have some great ideas, but I still feel as though it would be a touchy subject. Something inside of me feels guilty for not telling him everything that's going on, I really wish that I knew what the best way was to handle it all. Hopefully I'll figure it out in time.

Cruising through more mountainous roads I produce another joint from my pack of smokes. My brother lights it up for us immediately and asks me if I mind dropping him off at work at 3:00pm. He works at a competing grocery five minutes away from where I work, which is more acceptable for him seeing as how he is 16 years old. He'll be out of there in less than a year if my predictions are correct, which I'm sure they are.

  I pull into a convenience store just outside of town and run into to grab my brother two packs of smokes. He doesn't ask me to do this, and manages to get smokes on his own on a regular basis, but I figure while I have him here I might as well hook him up to make things easier. It's the right thing to do, and apparently the only thing beside a vehicle and a little weed that I can offer. He's really got shit lined up right.

  After taking a deliberately two hour drive back into town we arrive at his place of work. My brother reaches his hand out over the center console and waits for my subsequent shake before getting out of the car. He tells me to hit him up later when I have time and walks into the store ten minutes early.

26. Penance

Being forced to apologize for something that I believe in really bothers me. I don't even know where to begin. I'll never understand why people are so afraid of human emotion. I was angry, distraught, and frustrated. They should all be thanking me for not doing more damage. For stopping when I did, and not tearing the entire room apart or taking out one of the staff members that restrained me. I still had plenty of fight in me when they stuck their little sedation needle in my arm, but figured it would prolong my stay here, which is not something that I want to do. I sit here staring at an empty piece of paper with a pen in my hand, fighting the urge to draw stick figures all over it giving the middle finger. This all just seems so stupid.

I wish that I could hit fast forward and be done with this place entirely. Not for the sole reason to use again, but because I feel like a prisoner, and have felt that way ever since I got thrown into that police cruiser last Friday morning. I figured that I'd end up court ordered to rehab, because that's what they do. It's their little way of trying to clean up the streets.   A completely futile act if you ask me. I'm out here because I want to be, and until I don't want to anymore, it's where I am going to stay. My addiction is my life right now; I've already accepted that with open arms. Forcing me to stay away from it isn't going to change anything in the long run. That has to come from me – and I know that. One more week and I can feel free again. I just have to get though the next seven days.

Deciding to suck it up, and give in so that I can ultimately get out of here, I start writing my false apology. They never said that it had to be genuine. I'm supposed to present this to everyone today at the allotted time slot reserved for "patient presentations", right before "supper" as it says on the schedule. I can't wait for it to be over, not because I have to speak, but because I have to lie to everyone, when the only thing that I want to do is scream and yell all over again leaving a path of destruction in my wake. I have to keep my eye on the prize though. Get it over with, and get out of here. I finish my fabricated speech in all of 15 minutes and wait to be released from my slightly more comforting cell.

A staff member comes and releases me, and I head straight to the phones to call my brother. I need an update to see where everything is at. Since I can't receive calls here unless it's an emergency I have no way of knowing unless I initiate the call. I quickly dial his cell phone and wait for him to pick up anxiously. Voice mail. I leave a message telling him I'll call again in an hour. I'll get him then.

People are looking at me differently now, like I'm some sort of crazy person that needs to be locked up. Wary eyes purposefully look away when I get close, I pretend I don't notice. Ironically the same judgments that fly around on the outside amongst the "normal" people are exactly the same in here. As soon as you step outside of what is considered to be acceptable behavior – you are pinned as a threat, no matter what the setting. This makes me even more disturbed so I decide to glare back at anyone who gives me a funny look. There's nothing in the rules about that. The next seven days are going to suck, but there's nothing that they can do to keep me here once they are up. I yearn for the building to explode.

Lunch time comes and I sit by myself picking at the slop that came up from the cafeteria. Even the lunch meat itself looks like it should be fed to pigs rather than humans. I ate better living out of the truck, which is saying a lot. Treatment facilities are setup completely wrong, someday they'll get it right, I'll never see it, but at least it's a nice thought to have. Everyone around me is medicated beyond the point of even having a personality anymore. Even the hardest people are seen staring at inanimate objects and thanking random people for giving them trivial things like a pen or a glass of water. I can't accept this environment as a solution, and I'm surprised that I ever did in the past. With age comes wisdom I suppose, I just can't do this anymore, it makes no sense.

Lunch time is over, time for a smoke – or four. I'm still being ignored by everyone, and I don't care. The less people I have to deal with the better. I don't like any of them anyways. No friends to be made during this stint, which relieves me on so many levels. Friends in here always end up turning into more work in the long run. It's best to keep to yourself and not get wrapped up in the hype of "saving" someone. I'm certainly the wrong person for that role, and would be more detrimental than anything else to someone's recovery. Time to go back to the phones.

I find out from my brother that Nikki has managed to get out of the city completely. She found out what happened to me from a friend of ours on the streets who saw me get picked up by the police. This friend of ours decided to show up at the court during my little trial last Monday and managed to get all of the details, I had no idea he was in the public crowd of people, but hearing about it amuses me. He ends up all over the city, and has all kinds of useful information in his head, which he loves to hand out to the people that he trusts. Nikki's parents came out and fixed the truck so that she could make it back to our hometown where they set her up in a cheap apartment. She told my brother to tell me that she loves me, and that she'll be out to get me when the two weeks is up. That's a small load off of my mind.

I walk back to the common room and sit on chair mentally preparing myself for what I am about to do. At least the good news has cheered me up a bit, I'm just going to get this over with as quickly as possible, by 4:00pm I'll be done and getting ready to pick at more slop from downstairs. For the first time since I got here – I'm actually looking forward to "supper".

Everyone has congregated for patient presentation time, and I walk to the front of the room to stand behind the beat up wooden podium. A staff member by my side explains that I would like to apologize for my episode yesterday. This isn't true at all – apologizing is the last thing that I want to do – but I simply don't have a choice other than to go along with it. I pull a folded piece of white lined paper out of my pocket and place it on the podium. Looking up, and with much chagrin, I begin.

"I would like to take a moment to provide you all with an explanation for my actions yesterday during group. I have had ample time to ponder what I did, and still feel as though I was somewhat justified, but I shouldn't have taken it out on all of you. In truth – none of you are actually to blame, so my accusatory tone was wrong. For this I apologize. I would also like to assure everyone that I am indeed of sound mind and do not ever mean to cause any harm. I have strong feelings about certain things, and yesterday was just a result due to some of those things building up inside of me. I will do everything in my power to control myself in the future, and wish everyone here the best of luck as always. You only have to endure seven more days of me here, and then you can pretend as if I never even existed. Thank you for listening."

Broken applause trickled out of the crowd while most of the staff members looked at me with confused and shocked faces. Apparently they were expecting something else, I can't surmise what. That was the most genuine thing that I could come up with, and they should be sufficiently satisfied, at least I complied with their wishes. What more could they possibly want?

I stepped away from the podium calmly and began walking past everyone in the room in silence as they stared at me blankly. I could feel their eyes piling up on my back with each step that I made toward the door in the back of the room. I finally pushed the door open and felt a smile slowly stretch across my face – only one week left.

27. Alone

We have a problem. Brad has assisted in getting me into trouble once again, but this time it wasn't concerning the law. This time it concerns Dave and his fiance. This time my living situation has been put on the line. It seems that no matter how I slice it – Brad is always going to leave me holding the shit end of the stick. I need to come up with a plan, and quickly.

I came home from hanging with my brother to get ready for work and all kinds of shit went down. I walked right into the middle of a verbal battle between Dave and Brad. Brad acting ridiculous and defending his heroin use as if Dave has attacked his mother and Dave stacking my belongings up near the front door. At first it didn't all sink in. What could I have possibly done that would have persuaded Dave to kick me out of the house. Slowly it all started to make sense. Brad had thrown me under the bus, and clearly Dave was not cool with the heroin use. I took the queue saving my dignity, and apologized to Dave while tossing my shit in my car. He seemed a bit disturbed by my calmness, but it's his house, and I can't expect anyone to actually put up with it. I'm really bummed out about it and have no clue yet as to what I am going to do, but I'll figure something out.

Brad has a cousin across town that lives in the projects, I assume he's planning on going there, and I'm sure he won't mind if I stay there for a few nights, at least until I come up with another plan. Especially considering how he is the one who fucked everything up for me in the first place. I don't even bother getting into it with him. I don't see the point. I need to start distancing myself from Brad anyways, which I already been contemplating the last few days. He is bringing me right down with every single bad decision that he makes, and now I have lost my roommates. I hate this. I never should have even stuck that goddamn needle in my arm that night. He just wasn't happy until he had someone else to share his misery with. He just wanted to ruin one more life in order to make him feel better about fucking his own up.

We're done stuffing shit into my car and off to the projects. One step closer to having nothing, this cycle is spinning out of control quickly. I wasn't prepared for things to get this messed up so quickly, but I signed up for this – time to ride it out as best I can. We show up and carry what little possessions I have into the spare bedroom of the apartment, which is already cluttered with random junk. The whole place smells like bad cooking and dirty laundry. I have heard three different babies crying in random places throughout the building after only being here for about ten minutes. This is definitely one step lower than living at Dave's. The good thing about that is that it will give me plenty of motivation for getting out, I'll kill myself if I stay here too long – it can only be a temporary solution.

I pile up a bunch of clothes and blankets in the corner of the room and take a seat. Reaching into my bag I pull out the little wooden box and stare at it. Brad is standing in the doorway smiling. He doesn't care that we are here; it makes no difference to him at all. All he cares about it what's inside the box that I'm holding. I tell him to throw me the cordless phone. I dial work – again, and call myself out for the night, continuing with the fake cough skit. They don't believe me at all this time, but fuck them. I need some time to collect myself, and think about how I am going to get out of this mess.

Brad stares at me like a lap dog panting, and waiting to be fed. I pull out the works and start cooking up. At least I'll get him out of my face for now, and have some relief of my own. Cook, shoot, nod, done. I have entered the "land of make believe". Chasing my problems away with the brown elixir, I fall into a deep dreamless slumber.

Standing Room Only

Somewhere in the middle of the night I wake up and decide to be somewhat productive, grabbing a pen and paper to jot down some ideas on. I need a place to live. I need a different job. I need to surround myself with better people so as to help keep me on the right track. I need to stop using heroin. I immediately cross this point out with the pen that I am holding. I don't just cross it out though; I scribble it out until there's a giant black blotch in place of where the words used to be. This one scares me, and for some reason, it scares me more than anything else. I have barely even gotten into it, and it has a complete hold on me that I don't want to admit to. It has already caused so many problems in just this short amount of time; things are bound to get worse. I need to find a way to better manage it. I need to find a lasso that will actually fit around it and be strong enough to keep it in place. A lasso made out of thick twisted metal cable. A lasso made out of barbed wire. I really don't know how to accomplish this.

The sun slowly starts to shine through the window in the room as I am engulfed with an extreme sadness. I want this to all go away, and I want to start over 4 months ago knowing everything that I know right now. I want another chance, and I want to do things differently. But I can't. I can't change anything that has already happened, and the only thing I can control is my own future. I hunker into the corner and bury my face into my hands. I don't want anybody to see me like this, suffering, failing, and losing it all. I was really kidding myself. I can't believe that I actually thought I could keep this all together. I was nuts. I can't stop thinking about my family and how they are going to react if they ever find out what I am doing. I just can't think about anything right now without practically losing my mind. I feel as though I am having a mental break down. If I could I would stuff myself into the smallest box I could find, lock it, and have it tossed into the largest body of water that there is, just to keep me away from this horrible drug. Even then I fear that I would find a way to claw myself out and hold my breath for days until I surfaced, just to scour the earth for more, more, more. I want to be pulverized into a million minuscule pieces light years beyond any hope of repair. I want to have never existed in the first place, just to spare the ones around me of all the madness that is guaranteed to come due to this terrible addiction.

I roll over and lean up against the wall curling my arms around the backs of my knees. Desperately trying to fall back asleep I can feel myself fighting the urge to cry, which doesn't happen often. I shake my head furiously and force myself to keep it together. If one tear falls I know that I'll completely lose it and put my fist through the wall in front of me.

28. So Close

Three days have passed since my public apology. People have been leaving me alone for the most part. I think that most are anxious for my departure, I am as well. This experience was rougher than the others for some reason. Perhaps because I went into it knowing that I wasn't going to make any real progress. I have too many things to take care of and deal with before making that leap. I don't come from a rich family that can just send me away to a 90 day treatment facility and take care of me for years and years afterward so that I don't have to ever deal with anything that might lead me back to heroin. I need to get things pointed in the right direction at least before I can give in and fight this addiction from the inside. It's going to take everything I have to beat it, if I can beat it.

The system calls my addiction a disease – I disagree. In my eyes – the drug is the disease, and the addiction is a byproduct of that disease. Once you taste it – it has you. And before the addiction, comes the drug itself. Makes sense to me, and I don't think that anyone should be able to use the notion of disease as an excuse. Everyone here has consciously sought out their drug of choice and married it with the utmost commitment. That's not a disease. Leukemia is a disease. Alzheimer's is a disease. And these things infest innocent people who don't wake up every morning trying to find ways to facilitate them. To me it's a cop-out. I love heroin. End of story. It's my fault, and no amount of psychobabble in the world is going to make me believe different. This is why I am forever unsuccessful when forced to go this route.

In truth I don't have all of the answers, and I know that. If I did I wouldn't be in this situation, or at least that's what I'd like to believe. Regardless, I have four days left in this shithole and can't wait to get out. I'm going to be going back home, and shack up with my girl. Her parents have already paid the rent on her place three months in advance, knowing that she'd just lose it if they didn't. She grabbed a job right down the street at a small restaurant chain, I'm curious to see if she'll still have it by the time I get out, she doesn't have a very good track record with holding down employment. She's slightly worse than I am when it comes to dealing with authority. In a lot of ways she's completely out of her mind and unstable, which is one of the reasons why I love her. I don't really trust anyone who couldn't be considered at least a little crazy. I also don't find most people to be interesting at all, and would rather chew glass than spend more than five minutes listening to their boringness. It will be good to get home.

The counselors have given up on me, which I find comforting, I think that they know I'm not ready, and I'd rather be real about it with them then forced to fake it. I am grateful for this. I could easily be pushed to another episode if these people were so inclined, and I think that they all know that. Nobody has mentioned my apology. Not one single person. It's as if it never even happened. I think they're trying to forget about it. They never gave me any guidelines except for length, and never asked to see what I had prepared, so for the most part it's on them if it wasn't what they expected. The staff here should know better than to give someone like me free reign on anything – unless they are prepared for all possible results. Personally I think that it's funny. These people are amazing at sweeping shit under the carpet rather than actually dealing with it, which is extremely contradictory to everything that this place stands for – in my opinion. Everything is kept at arm's length, because when it's in your face – it's scary and uncomfortable. Fear rules all, outside and inside, doesn't matter where you are or who you are with. A clear line can easily be drawn to separate the fearless and the afraid. The fearless are few and constantly trying to recruit new members, while on the other side of the line there's standing room only. More and more people join every single second stuffing themselves in next to others who hunker down and let them through without confrontation or protest, while the fearless scream for them to come back and hold strong, but inevitably the wrong side keeps growing and growing like a landfill that has overcome its space. I'll never join the afraid.

I talked to my brother again the other day – he offered to come get me when my time here is up, but I told him that Nikki will be fine running down, and that we'd come right back. I didn't tell him that we are going to make a quick stop first to grab some shit, but I assume he already figures that. He doesn't pressure me unless he thinks it's necessary, which has happened in the past, but he knows that otherwise I'm going to do what I want and nothing is going to stop me. He's the only one who understands that enough to respect it, and I honestly can't comprehend how, I'd never expect anyone to respect my actions, but he does. He never got involved in anything like I have when it comes to drugs. I guess he had a good example in his life by watching me fuck up at every turn because of them, but even still he was able to stay away from them, and not be as stupid as I have been. I'm glad about that; I wouldn't wish this life on anyone, and certainly not someone that I care about. I'm glad that I still have him in my corner though, sometimes it feels like there really isn't anyone else there, which I completely understand.

I also called my Mother this morning, who was very upset, but she held it together for the most part on the phone, I'm sure she's a complete mess right now. I hate what I have done to her by living this way. I've literally put her through hell. I've dragged her through the flames and turned around to empty a gas can on her burning corpse. At least that's what it feels like in my stomach when I think about the pain and suffering that I have put her through. She doesn't deserve it, and none of it was ever intentional. It's hard for me to even talk to her at times because I can hear the anguish in her voice. I can feel the strain through the phone that she is forcing down her throat when she speaks. It tears me up inside, and makes me feel like the worst person on the planet. I never meant to cause anybody anything, but I have. That doesn't even include the rest of my family, it's all too much for me to even think about, ultimately that will be the only way that I'll be able to get off this shit – is for them, not me. Fuck.

My plan is to hit the road when these four days are up, grab some good shit to bring back with us, and pick up some sort of bullshit job at another nearby grocery store back home. At least then I can generate some cash on a regular basis and try to get back into the swing of things - one step closer toward the possibility of living a "normal" life. A life that doesn't include me climbing out of a truck bed every morning and running from the cops every couple of hours. A life that includes changing my clothes more frequently than every 3-5 days. A life that doesn't force me to have eyes in the back of my head constantly running surveillance to make sure that I'm not going to get jumped and robbed by the other degenerates, like myself, who are desperate and roaming the streets. A life that actually has the possibility of sustaining life – I am convinced that if things stay like this, I'll be dead within the next six months.

29. Safety

I walk into work for the first time in awhile, the weekend has come and I'm on the day shift. The glares from my supervisors are piercing to say the least; I can feel the light from their eyes stabbing me from every direction. They all have their theories, and I'm certain that most of them end in termination of employment. I'll ride things out for as long as I can, if that's what ends up happening in the long run then so be it. For right now the only thing I can do is show up and see what happens. So that's what I'll do. I don't really care except I hate going through the process of finding a new job. If I could somehow manage to make enough money without working – that's exactly what I'd do. But I haven't figured that out yet.

I stare at each new "number" that enters my line wondering if there is anything even remotely interesting about them. Usually I can tell right away that there isn't. Every so often one of them displays a glimmer of hope, but you never can really tell without actually talking, and I don't ever bother doing that. Beep, Beep, Beep. I hope I do get fired, that way I don't have to even deal with telling them that I quit.

Break time finally comes and I once again rush outside to smoke as much as I possibly can. My supervisor catches me on the way back into the store and asks me how I'm feeling. I tell her better, and realize that she is making her own assessments based on how I look and act. Thankfully there's no drug testing that goes on here, I bet they all wish that policy existed. Then again they'd lose half of their work force and never be able to find anyone to perform these menial tasks. It all works out in the end.

I plod through the next couple of hours focusing on getting out and manage to still have my mind by the time I leave. I still need to figure things out in order to rectify my current living situation. I can't stay at Brad's cousin's apartment, it will never work. I'm not even sure I'll be able to do it tonight – last night was bad enough. I need to call Kristen when I get to a phone. I decide to stop at a pay phone so that I can make this call without Brad even knowing my whereabouts for the night. I really hope that she can help me out. I have an excuse to go over there too, because I have to nail that paper for her, which should only take me about an hour anyways. She answers the phone questioningly, and then cheers up immediately as soon as she hears the sound of my voice. She's glad to hear from me, and so soon. I tell her a little bit about my current situation and she is overjoyed to help me out, especially since it will just be me. I tell her I'll be over in an hour or so and hang up.

Running up the stairs to Brad's cousin's apartment, I couldn't be happier to know that I won't be sleeping here again. I grab what little belongings I even bothered to bring in from the car the night before and split up the dope that's left to leave for Brad. I shove it in his pants pocket where he'll find it when he comes to his senses. He's already ripped out of his mind and snoring away on the couch as usual. His cousin is locked up in her room with the TV blaring – high on whatever prescription drugs she could get her hands on for the day.

I'm out the door and down the stairs almost as quickly as I climbed them. Off to Kristen's for a night of normalcy, and some secret telling. Kristen has always been extremely tolerable of anything that I get myself into. She has always been a straight shooter, but finds my glaringly opposing choices to be intriguing, and therefore puts up with pretty much anything I throw at her. It's a weird relationship, and one that also includes some extra physical benefits as well. This is going to be a fun night. I just really hope that she doesn't feel like I am taking advantage of her, I know that she won't, but it's something that concerns me nonetheless.

She greets me at the door with a gigantic hug and kiss on the lips, apparently very happy to see me. I immediately decide to keep the heroin conversation for another day, perhaps tomorrow. I don't want to ruin tonight, especially after seeing her reaction to my arrival. It's best that we both enjoy the night and not taint it with the drug addiction conversation. I will however tell her, and soon, I have never been able to actually keep anything from Kristen, it's always felt really wrong to lie to her or withhold any kind of pertinent information. Besides, she already knows that something serious is going on, that's why I'm here, and that's why she had to come bail me out a few days ago with the car situation. She also knows that I'll come clean and tell her, yet none of this affects her mood toward me, because she genuinely likes me as a person and is an actual real friend. In truth she is the most real friend I have, and has been the absolute best friend out of any acquaintance I have ever had. I truly hope that I never do anything to harm our bond, that's my biggest concern of all. It would kill me if I ever did something to hurt her.

We swiftly go inside and have a seat on the couch. I pull out a joint, which she doesn't partake in, but has no problem with me smoking at all. We've done this before. She lifts up the remote and kills the TV, then points another one at the stereo she has setup in the corner and flicks it on. This is also standard procedure for our little gatherings. We're going to be here talking for quite some time. I suspect that we'll start making our way toward bed somewhere around 3:00am, and I don't have to work tomorrow, so we'll spend the day together as well.

Kristen has always been somewhat infatuated with me; ever since the first time that we met back in middle school when she moved here. Ironically I used to give her shit and make fun of her a lot during those years, but never in a malicious manner, that's just how our relationship was at the time. As the years went on we grew closer and closer, almost without having a choice. We found that we both agreed with each others views on a lot of important issues, which also made for some terrific discussions over the years. This is part of the glue that keeps us together, however I am quite certain that she has much deeper feelings for me and wishes that we could be together on some level. I have always just considered her my absolute best friend, with some other benefits as well, but I don't think that it would be a good idea for us to start anything too serious for some reason. Even though we have a lot in common, we do certainly also have our difference, and those differences are very different.

Tonight is going to be great, I need this, and I'm sure she needs it on some level as well. It's been a long time, and the little trip the other night doesn't count. We hunker down on our respective seats on the couch and begin our relaxing night together.

30. Out

Nikki is waiting in the parking lot when I finally exit the building that has been my prison for the last two weeks. I am overjoyed when I finally get in the passenger seat of my former residence. Nikki looks great, but is clearly still using just as much as before. The only difference being that she is no longer living in the back of a truck. She can tell by the look on my face that I want to go score immediately, and has already come prepared with a descent stack of cash, which I assume came from her parents. I can also tell that she was hoping that I'd want to score, as she clearly wants to bring home as much shit as we can get our hands on. Her motives are crystal clear.

She seems happy to see me, but not quite as happy as I would have expected. After a quick hug and kiss, she starts immediately telling me everything that sucks – like I'm back to clean up all of the issues. I don't really understand this, and can tell that we are going to have a verbal battle soon if she keeps acting this way. I try to remind myself that I haven't gotten high in weeks and that she is strung out on whatever she can get her hands on. I ignore her ranting and tell her to bring me to the spot so I can score.

It feels good, but yet a little strange to be making this walk up the familiar path to the front door of the old tattered house. I have the weird sense that people are watching me from all around, waiting to pounce like a wild agile cat. I assume that this is due to the past few weeks, and try brushing it off as best I can. The exchange occurs, and the usual guy looks at me oddly, realizing that he hasn't seen me around in awhile. He also seems a bit apprehensive as if I am working for someone or something. Finally he shakes his head quickly from side to side and finishes our transaction, obviously realizing that he was wrong. I head back to the truck.

Out

What happened out here while I was gone? It's like the world has turned itself upside down and gotten even weirder overnight. I don't like it, but I have no choice but to return, and I certainly don't want to be back in rehab or jail, so this seems like a much better alternative. The people look different. The cars look different, even the streets themselves look different. It hasn't been that long though. I don't understand. I'm going to not think about it and focus on getting home. I am anxious to see Nikki's new place, it will be great to feel as though we have an actual home to go to. That is a feeling that will once again be completely new to me, and I'm sure very odd.

Nikki is itching to get high the minute she knows that I'm holding the good stuff from our favorite dealer. I tell her to get us home first. She doesn't like that, but I insist anyways. She can lose her mind with madness – I don't care. I'm the one that has been clean for two weeks and is dying for a fix, she's been using right along, and can wait 45 minutes until it's actually safe to shoot up. Sometimes she is completely unreasonable and gets extremely miserable whenever she doesn't get her own way. Once again – I don't care.

We get to the new place of residence, after a tension filled drive that seemed as though it took forever. The new apartment seems really nice. It's on the first floor with one neighbor upstairs. It's furnished with hard wood floors throughout and tall ceilings. I particularly like the sliding wood doors that separate each room from the next; they add a nice touch to the overall atmosphere of the place. It's a one bedroom apartment, but the rooms are rather large giving plenty of comfortable space. The little furniture that we do suddenly have seems completely swallowed up by each massive area – very cool. I'm surprised that her parents set her up with such a cool place, I was expecting something small in one of the many projects that are scattered throughout the city. This was anything but. We are close to downtown which will make transportation a cinch, because Nikki can simply walk to the restaurant that she works at during the day. I can in turn take the truck if and when I do find a job. Aside from her obvious impatience to use, things seem to have taken a very positive turn. This is something that I can work with.

After checking the place out I sit down on the new donated couch and pull the familiar packet out of my pocket. I already feel the heat traveling from my fingers and down the length of my arm just from holding it. The anticipation is monumental. Making this leap once again to my secret lover is a tougher decision that I had originally thought. I carefully tear it open at the corner, nonetheless, and get ready to cook. Nikki has already retrieved all of the tools necessary to perform this little ritual, obviously not taking my recent recovery into consideration at all. She doesn't care; she just wants her fix, like a good little addict.

I set her up with a shot first, because I need a minute to really stare at mine. Before I can even properly hand it to her she has it stuck into her arm as a small breathy sigh escapes her lips. Now it's my turn. I cook myself a small safe amount since my tolerance is completely gone – this is why most people overdose. I fill up the needle and take a bit of time to really reflect on what I'm about to do. In this one little dose, I'm going to throw it all away – willingly. All the pain and suffering from detox, all the control and willpower that I was forced to display for the last two weeks – gone, in just this one little shot. At least I know that I'm capable of doing it. That just means that I can do it again in the future. I kiss the clear plastic tubing before the needle, and plunge it into my vein – just like old times.

The intensity of the rush is almost enough to completely knock me off of my feet. There's something particularly special about this session – due to drying out – it's just like using heroin for the very first time. That's the one benefit to relapse; the first few weeks are euphoric beyond explanation. As if there was ever a "hook" needed to keep the addiction going – this is one of those hooks. This is the feeling that you are forever chasing day after day as soon as you have used for the first time. You don't want the feeling to ever disappear, you want to lock it up in the most secure thing you can find, and not let anyone else have it. You want it to be yours to control and access at all times, and at a moment's notice. You want to feel this way forever. The only catch is that you can't, and you don't. The feeling itself levels out after awhile and you need the poison in order to survive – In order to keep your body from tearing you apart on the inside. That's when the pleasure starts to dissipate and the depression of your lifestyle takes over. I've done this many times now, and still run right back to doing it all over again, knowing full well exactly what the outcome will be every single time, only hoping that each time I will once again cheat the ultimate bottom – death. Even with death being a serious complication, and possibility, I still find myself unable to resist the sweet taste of my favorite substance on earth.

For now I have much to enjoy, and another few days to really ride the experiences that are so rich and fulfilling when using this dangerous drug. I'll try to take it slow this time, and ultimately get things figured out. I'm in a completely different setting now, and at least have a much better chance at success, whether or not I'll fuck it all up again is entirely up to me.

31. Normalcy

Kristen and I had a wonderful night together, and this morning I told her what has been going on. I also told her that I am taking steps toward getting things back in line, step one: stay away from Brad as much as possible. She was very happy with that fact alone, so much so I think it helped her to cope with the fact that I can now be considered a heroin addict. She didn't already know exactly what was going on, but she had had a pretty good idea that it was along these lines. She thought something drug related, or a problem with the law. Given my track record neither one would be considered a stretch, so she was prepared for the worst, and knew that before agreeing to let me camp out her place. This made me feel a thousand times better, because I would never use Kristen like that, and wanted her to understand that fully. It seemed as though she did, and I will never be able to thank her enough.

We decide to go check out some of our favorite places a few towns over. There's an artsy type town that we used to go visit back in the day when life was much easier and less complicated. Today seemed like a perfect day to take off and enjoy ourselves. I of course need to medicate a little bit before we do, but I am planning on only using a little bit, just to keep the cravings at bay. I have no interest in nodding in and out of consciousness today with Kristen, and I don't want to be a burden on her in any way. I run upstairs to the bathroom and lock the door behind me. It's really weird to have any of this stuff out in the open in front of someone who doesn't use, I have no idea why really, but it just is. I guess because it's not something that I am proud of at all, and I don't want the people that I care about to even see these things in reality. I cook a small amount, and take a hit that will be safe and manageable.

Normalcy

Back downstairs I see that Kristen is ready to hit the road and smiling at me with her beautiful teeth always showing. She's very proud of her teeth, and makes it a point to smile perfectly; I usually mimic it back to get a quick laugh out of her – and to mess her up. She's a fun girl.

We jump in her car and head out of town, picking up coffees on the way. Kristen doesn't smoke, but doesn't mind if I do in her car. She really is beyond accommodating; most people are assholes about that. I just hope that someday I can be as good of a friend to her as she has been to me; I doubt that day will ever come though, for the most part, I don't really have anything too productive to offer – unless of course somebody needs advice on breaking the law in multiple ways. Evading police is a useful skill to have; I could probably give some good pointers there. Kristen will never need any of these skills though – that's ok, I have a paper to write.

As we drive I am feeling really good about things. I still have no plan for living on my own – there is no way that I could swing it by myself with my current salary. I would first have to find a real job, and I don't see that happening any time soon. I'll figure something out eventually. The trees drift by the car in a controlled blur that makes me smile. I peek at Kristen who is focused on the road like the diligent driver that she is, she sees me smiling, and bares her teeth once again. I'm once again reminded of how glad I am to be here.

We show up to the old faithful parking lot that we always used in the past to drop the car and continue throughout the city on foot. It's a mere dollar to leave it here for the afternoon, perfect. Some things never change, which is extremely comforting. Out on the street the air smells fresh and cool, different from back home, more alive. I throw my arm around Kristen's waist and she leans closer into me. She is wearing a light suede coat that I catch a whiff of every so often mixed with the faint scent of her fruity shampoo. Love the fresh smell of a woman – for a minute it takes my mind off of the heroin.

Browsing the stores with Kristen is fun as she always shows me interesting things and wants to know what I think about everything. Sharing a lot of the same odd interests heightens the entire experience. My buzz is holding strong and the cravings are sufficiently satisfied for the time being. Things are perfect. If only I could freeze time – these are the days that I am always looking for in life. This is all I ever really ask for. Other than times like this with people that I can actually tolerate; there's isn't really anything else that I want. I just want to be left alone to do my own thing with whoever I want or by myself if I wish. I don't want to give all of my time to a grocery store for 40 fucking dollars a night. That's the most perfect definition of insanity in my opinion. Somehow there has to be a better way to live, and actually attain a lifestyle that makes sense.

The place that we go to eat at is nice, and it's the same place that we always used to go to anytime that we came here. For some unknown reason the food is exceptionally good here and affordable at the same time. The atmosphere is really nice, and the people leave you alone for the most part, not pestering you with specials and useless shit. I like that. After a nice lunch we decide to head back to her house, and maybe just chill out and watch a movie together. She'll be going back to work in the morning – she's a normal person with a normal job so she works during the day all week and has the weekends off. It's a schedule that I wouldn't mind having; then again there isn't really an ideal work schedule in my opinion – unless that schedule includes not working at all.

Kristen's job expects her to be there at 7:30 in the morning, so she'll want to actually get some sleep tonight, which essentially leaves me to my own devices in the morning. She doesn't have a problem with me staying here alone, and sees it as company for her two cats anyways. I'm going to nail the paper tomorrow while she is at work, that way she doesn't have anything to worry about there, and I will at least be somewhat of a contribution, even though that's something I already owe her from her hook up the other night. Regardless I need to find something nice to do for her on my own, she has all but saved me, twice now, and I need to stay focused on not fucking things up.

We pop in one of our favorite thought provoking movies and curl up on the couch together under a blanket. Within an hour or so Kristen is fast asleep, so I decide to finish out the movie before waking her up and bringing her upstairs. I'm a bit tired as well, and can't wait to go lay down next her. The movie finally finishes and I manage to get her in my arms before she opens her eyes on the way up the stairs. She doesn't say anything, just lights the way with those shiny white teeth. Once I set her down gently on the bed, she falls back asleep in seconds. I change out of my clothes and curl up next to her looking forward to a peacefully and fulfilling night of sleep.

32. Restart

It's back to reality as I notice that it's about 11:00am already. I slept like a rock last night. It felt so good to not be sleeping in an institution. Nikki is still out, and I suddenly wonder if she was supposed to work today. She hasn't even mentioned her job to me, I'm not even sure that she knows I'm aware of it. I get out of bed and notice immediately that my muscles are aching. Getting used to the heroin again might take some time. I'm prepared. I walk into the kitchen to see if we have the necessary ingredients for coffee, and begin to think about applying for a job. I haven't worked in months, and the idea of going back couldn't be less appealing, but I have to do something now that I have actually been given a second chance. Money is a necessity unless I want to end up back in the truck again living in parking lots.

There's a small coffee pot, which I assume someone left here, sitting on the counter. It looks very used and old, but I don't care. I rummage through the cupboards trying to find a filter. There aren't any. I doubt that there's any actual coffee anyways, so I throw on my coat and some shoes and decide to talk a walk to find some. It feels like I have been gone from this place for years, it'll be good to get reacquainted with things again. It's brisk outside, but not too bad once you get walking, I head toward a chain coffee shop about half of a mile away. Not much has changed since I was last here. Incidentally my new apartment is about two streets over from Dave's house, so I'm back in the exact same neighborhood as before. I notice no new signs or businesses, and everything literally looks exactly as I left it. For some reason this disturbs me, and I can't quite figure out why.

The normal "during the day" actions are going on around me as I notice a group of high school kids walking to a local pizza shop for lunch. They saunter about without a care in the world; I wish I could tell them how it's really all going to turn out, but I wouldn't want to scare the little fuckers. The cars are still annoying as ever, people blowing their horns at every little thing, speeding around as if they are always late to wherever they are going. Time passes, but nothing ever really changes.

I grab myself the biggest coffee I can afford with the loose change that I found on the counter before I left. Back out on the street I remember the grocery store that is another five minute walk from here – I head in that direction. I'll put in an application and try to get a position stocking shelves rather than working a register. I just want something that will allow me to work at my own pace and without the strange interaction with the public. I think that I'll be able to tolerate that much better than waiting on my constant flow of "numbers" who do nothing but annoy me. I hope they have something like that available.

On the way over I think about whether or not I'll be able to manage the addiction this time in a manner that will keep me from losing it all over again. I wonder if I can find a way to not use as much as I did, and keep myself on a more even keel. Nikki's use has obviously done nothing but gotten worse since I got picked up. That's going to make things difficult and build tension between us. This time is going to be weird, I have an odd feeling about it, but for some reason deep down inside, I think I can do it. Maybe that's just me being delusional in hoping that I'll still be able to bed down with my favorite substance every night without it being a problem. Maybe I'm just in denial. I don't know.

I walk into the busy grocery store and walk to the service desk for an application. The 20 year old girl behind it flashes me a smile, and I ask her for the paperwork. She gives me a blank form and tells me to fill it out. I find a bench in the corner of the store and start working on it so that I can bring it right back. When I get to the phone number section I give them my brother's cell phone, I'll have to call him and let him know to be on the lookout in case they call – I have no phone, and no other means of contact. I check off a stocking position as my preference and bring the completed application back to the little girl behind the counter. She takes it smiling, and I head for the door.

That was easy, and I actually feel like I did something productive for the day. On my way back to the apartment I stop at a pay phone and fill my brother in. He tells me he'll let me know if hears anything and that he'll swing by in a couple of days when he's free. It's good to be back.

I walk into the apartment and can hear Nikki in the bathroom throwing up. I run across the kitchen to see what's going on and find her kneeling down in front of the toilet dry heaving.

"What's wrong?" I ask.

"I don't know. I just feel like shit. Woke up out of a sound sleep and headed straight to the toilet. I barely made it in time."

I find this to be a little odd, but have no reason to suspect anything unusual. I have noticed that she looks thinner than she did two weeks ago. I just figured it was the incessant drug use. She needs to take better care of herself, and she definitely needs to slow down on the dope. The fire in her eyes yesterday afternoon was fierce; I've seen that look before on my own face in the bathroom mirror - it's not a good place to be. I need to have a talk with her as soon as I think she'll actually take me seriously. When it comes to the drug itself, an addict is usually extremely defensive toward anything or anyone that tries to attack it. If I said anything to her about it right now, with the state that she's in, a small war would ensue. Sometimes it's not the actual person that you are talking to, but instead the drug incarnate. There is no chance of a reasonable conversation when this is the case. I'll wait patiently until the time is right.

"So are you working today?" I ask, nervous to hear the answer.

"I was supposed to be there at 9:00, they are just going to have to wait until I can stop puking my guts out." She yells back annoyed.

I take it that she has no intentions of letting them know that she won't be in today. As I had already thought, this job is not going to last. I believe that she has worked a total of about two months in the last four years or so, according to what she has told me at least. She is going to make keeping this apartment very difficult, especially if she wants to keep using the amount of drugs that she's on every day. Everything is going to go downhill, and quickly. I can already tell. Nikki is one of those people that when given anything manages to dig herself an even deeper hole. She's worse than I am when it comes to self destruction, which is saying a lot if you ask me. I tell her that I'm going to take the truck for a bit and visit a few people that I haven't seen in awhile. There's certainly no point in me sticking around here.

33. Push

I hear Kristen's soft footsteps as she moves around the room with calculated precision. A faint fruity smell fills the room as the steamy air from her recent shower wafts in behind her. She's being quiet on purpose for my benefit. She's trying to not wake me up as she gets ready for work. She really is a magnificent person. I slowly drift in and out of sleep while listening to her movements, mentally following her around the upstairs until I hear the front door close. I am guessing that it's somewhere around 7:00am, and decide to enjoy her fading scent in the bed a little longer.

Around 8:30am I wake up for real, and seek out coffee, which I am certain Kristen will have all the makings for, as she always does. Once the coffee is brewing, I start to relax and think about what I am going to do all day. I'm not used to being alone, but I like it. Some people really need to fill up all of their free time with mindless activities or constant human interaction in order to feel comfortable. I have never understood it - I do just fine on my own, and usually prefer it depending on the situation. It's nice to not have Brad up my ass every waking minute either. I really needed a break from him.

The really cool thing about me staying here is that I am basically completely off the map. Nobody would ever come looking for me here, except for my brother, and that's fine. I am planning on giving him a heads up soon anyways, I just can't figure out what reason I am going to give him for why I am here and suddenly not living at Dave's. Otherwise, however, I am hidden to the rest of the world. Brad for example has absolutely no way to find me. He doesn't even know where Kristen lives, and certainly doesn't have her phone number. This was my main goal when trying to figure out where to go. If he knew where I was he'd be knocking down my door the minute he ran out of dope to go get some more. I have decided to take those matters into my own hands, and will be making solo trips to the golden city from now on. I realize that this increases the dangers of it all, but bringing Brad with me has become more dangerous so I am left without a choice. I am going to go find him in a day or two and let him know what my plans are, he'll have to agree with me or he won't be able to score the good shit and at the price we get it at. I'll go down and pick it up, then bring it back home, deliver his cut, and then we disperse from there. That's my new plan.

The coffee pot increases its popping noises and speed – the signal that it's almost ready. I grab the cup I used the night before from the strainer by the sink and wait the last minute or so anxiously. The need for a fix is starting to creep up on me quickly. Luckily I have no place in particular to be today, and I'm left with the entire house to myself, with nobody to bother me at all. This is a very ideal situation. I pour the first cup of coffee and make my way into the living room. The small wooden box is upstairs in my backpack – waiting for me. I sit on the couch and try not to think about it – I don't want to give in yet. I flip on the TV as a distraction and start downing the coffee. It's 8:49am. The TV isn't helping. I can hear the wooden box rustling around in my bag trying to break itself free. I set down my coffee and all but run up the stairs.

I'm concerned about my addiction now, more than I have been in the past few weeks. I'm starting to see elements of Brad inside myself when it comes to the drug. The control that it seems to have over me is more powerful than a team of oxen dragging 40,000 pounds of steel blocks through the mud. I don't know if I will ever have the ability to stop. Eventually this shit is going to kill me. These are thoughts that I have as I pull everything out of the wooden box one by one and set them on the coffee table. All of the necessary tools are out and ready to go, all I have to do is implement. I get right to it shaking some of the brown dust into the metal cap, an electric shock travels through my body and I can't wait to feel it in my veins. There is nothing around me anymore, I could be sitting on a rock beside the ocean - the only concern I have right now is the mixture that is being sucked up inside my needle. I want it so bad that I can taste it in the back of my throat. I want it more than life itself in this very moment.

I pull in a deep breath and brace myself for the rush. It feels like I have entered a million different heavens all at once. The euphoria is almost too much for me to handle. My head is filled with air and my entire body is levitating in midair. New sensations that I have never felt before start to slowly take hold. My muscles begin turning to the consistency of glue and my chest feels like an elephant is standing on it. At first I don't understand and just figure these new sensations are from taking it easy over the past couple of days. Then a small twinge of panic sets in as I realize that I took too much. I somehow need to focus before it's too late. I stand up and immediately fall backwards on to the couch. The dizziness overpowers me. The room is spinning out of control – this is going to be difficult. Slowly rising again I steady myself against the coffee table using every muscle in my body. I just need to get my legs to cooperate now. It feels like I am walking on noodles as I make my way into the kitchen. So far I'm still conscious and I don't feel like I am dying. I'm not sure what dying feels like though so who knows. I make my way to the fridge and open it slowly – this action seems to take hours. The concept of time has disappeared completely from my head. I pull out a bottle of water and fumble with the cap until I finally get it open. I feel intense heat all over my body, and need to find a way to cool down. I need to make my way back to the couch, but anticipate that the next few hours are going to be extremely difficult. I reach down and open up the cabinet where Kristen keeps her alcohol and pull out a brand new bottle of vodka to bring back with me, I'm going to need something to stay awake.

Days have passed in my head, but the clock reads 9:22am. I have a long way to go before any of this starts to let up. Without seeking medical attention the effects from a non-fatal overdose can last quite awhile. If anything really bad was going to happen I think that it already would have, but I can't be completely certain. Each movement requires extreme effort to facilitate, and I have never felt like this before. It's not painful, at least not at the moment; instead it's actually peaceful beyond comprehension however I know that something is wrong. I need to sit down. I need to focus on staying awake. I need to have a smoke.

I sit and smoke until I run out of cigarettes. The clock reads 11:08am, and I'm surprised that time has bothered to move at all. I have completely given up on time at this point, just accepting the imprisonment that has occurred inside my head. Fighting it will only make matters worse, so I try not to think about it as I sit here staring at nothing and doing nothing. I wonder how many times Brad has pushed himself to this limit. I wonder if this is where he was mentally every time I'd find him on the couch completely incapacitated. I really have to be careful not to do this again. I have gotten lucky so far today and am still alive by some miracle, but luck is not something that I can bank on in the future. The possibilities of fatality are very real, and I just got my first actual reminder.

34. News

I spent the day seeing the few people that have decided to stay in my life despite my addiction. One really good friend of mine named Evan lives in the same town that my Mom does. I spend a few hours there hanging out, but not without a price. Evan informs me that a friend of mine from the artsy town that Kristen and I like to frequent a few times a year has died from a heroin overdose. I don't take the new information very well. I never do. No matter how many times death stares me in the face; I can't handle a friend dying from this shit. It also doesn't make me want to stop – it makes me want to use more. It's the only way that I can think of to deal with the immense pain from it all. I realize that I use heroin as an escape, but I don't care. I have to escape. Otherwise I'll die from sheer misery alone.

Tomorrow night a group of people who knew him are all planning on getting together and holding a vigil in the local park. I plan on attending. I'll see if Nikki could be bothered to go, but I doubt she will. That's fine with me; I'd rather go alone anyways. I really don't know what to do. Everything sucks right now, and it's supposed to be getting better. I'm supposed to be finding ways to stay off of the streets and actually maintain a somewhat productive lifestyle, even if it's only for me. I don't even see how that is attainable right now, and all the rehab in the world couldn't get me there. I need something else, but have no idea what it could possibly be.

In a stupor I drive back to the apartment, ready to use immediately when I get there. I don't feel good about this, but I also feel like I don't have a choice. The sadness that I'm feeling hurts more than anything else, and I have to find a way to medicate it before it destroys me. I can't keep losing people that matter to me, and losing someone from heroin especially hurts. I feel lower than dirt continuing to use while people are dying from exactly what I am doing. What the fuck is wrong with me? Have I become that heartless and cowardly? I feel like shit, and find myself running into the house to find a needle. Any needle. Just to make this pain go away.

Nikki is nodding off on the couch, which I am actually really happy about. I won't even have to deal with her in this instant. It can wait until I have dealt with myself and gotten some relief. A conversation with her right now would certainly put me over the edge, and I'd probably end up having a mental breakdown right here on the floor. Filled with a new found joy from having a clear path to my dope, I run to the closet and pull out the faithful little wooden box once again. I am extremely cautious as I measure out just enough so that I don't overdo it. The lack of tolerance will take a little while to build back up again – the tiniest bit too much could surely be a fatal dose. I need to dole it out to myself slowly, and carefully.

Once my shot is ready I take it immediately. I put the wooden box back and lay down on the bed staring at the ceiling. I am staring to feel slightly better as the focus in my mind drifts away from my dead friend for a moment. I stop thinking completely. The white detailing on the ceiling seems to be getting closer to my face with every second that passes. I follow the swirly designs and pick up on every spot of discoloration that litters the pattern. Breathing slow and steady – nothing matters right now. The drone of the radio coming from the living room has turned into white noise that constantly plays in my head with no beginning or end. It's as if someone has turned out the lights inside of me. I want to cry, but I can't. I want to change, but I can't. I want to save everyone, but I can't. I just can't. That's what I should change my name to – Can't. Apostrophe and all. It's certainly fitting.

I roll around in the bed all by myself for a long time and keep my mind off of anything that could possibly cause further distress. Once I come down, I'll have to deal with everything all over again – that's a guarantee – so there's no point in stressing about it now.

35. Love

Hands on my shoulders, I think. My tunnel vision desperately tries to focus on Kristen's face. I have no idea where I am or how I got there. She's talking but I can barely hear her muffled words. I think I'm still alive, but I can't be completely sure. My last memory is of me sitting on the couch staring off into space trying to wait out the large dose of heroin that I had shot. I wonder if it's still the same day or not. It must be. My hearing slowly starts to fade back in and I realize that Kristen is in a panic trying to make sure that I'm ok. I slowly start to realize what this all must look like. I'm apparently on the floor in between the couch and the coffee table. I don't remember picking up the needle or the wooden box so they must be in plain view somewhere. And then there's the bottle of vodka that is probably standing up on the floor near me.

Kristen starts pulling me to my feet and I do everything that I can to assist her, with the help of the coffee table I end up landing on the couch. I just need to figure out how to speak again so that I can explain everything to her. I certainly don't want her to panic and take matters into her own hands. Obviously I am going to come through this without any help from the outside, which has me quite relieved. I just have to let her know what happened.

"I...took....too much. I'll be...fine...soon." I manage to mumble.

She looks at me with worry and concern painting her features. I can tell that she understands though as she reaches down to take off her shoes. I close my eyes and feel the dope just starting to wear off as the pain is slowly creeping into my muscles. The ironic thing about overdosing on heroin is that there is no pain, until it's over. If you overdose to the point that Brad did a few weeks ago, and get woken up by that magical shot they give you at the hospital, everything immediately hurts like hell. Your respiratory system which was inches from shutting down is suddenly jolted to life and restored to normal functionality. All of the muscles that you have managed to numb so well are suddenly able to feel everything all at once. The same thing happens without that magical shot, the only difference being is that the process itself is slower, and the pain is prolonged. I have no idea what this is going to feel like, but I know already that I'm not going to like it. That's why I have the bottle of vodka ready, I'm sure I'm going to need it very soon. My breathing has moved one step up from extremely labored to slightly labored, and my lungs are beginning to feel like they are on fire. My stomach is rolling over inside of me and has a stabbing sensation every couple of minutes that renders me unable to move. My head is pounding and only getting worse. I felt none of this all day long, and anticipate a horrible night.

Kristen continues to stare at me like I am going to die at any moment. I must look horrible. I can't believe that I have managed to make this happen right here in her house. I never wanted her to see me like this. That fact alone has me just as upset as I am about the oncoming physical pain. Physical pain goes away eventually. Fuck. I can feel another wave of fatigue pin me to the corner of the couch. I attempt to reach for the bottle on the floor – Kristen understands and gets it for me. She opens it up, breaking the seal on the cap, and carefully hands it to me. I take a sip and cringe at the burn as it slides down my throat. The alcohol will only be so effective, but it's still light years better than not having anything to help dull the pain. I wish I could just have another hit, but I know that's completely out of the question.

Lifting the bottle to my lips once more I realize, for the first time, that my fingertips have started to turn blue. Apparently my circulation has been compromised in some way. Oh well, one more thing to worry about I guess. I guess that explains on some level the horrified looks that Kristen keeps giving me. I have really freaked her out, and I'm not happy about that at all. I feel like such a failure. Kristen asks me if I want anything to eat or drink from the kitchen, I just shake my head. She walks into the kitchen, clearly not wanting to leave me alone in fear that something is going to happen any second. I lie down on the couch and brace myself for the coming onslaught of discomfort.

The room starts to spin out of control, and I can tell that I am going to be sick very soon.

"I'm going to....puke." I tell Kristen desperately.

She runs to the kitchen and grabs a basin from under the sink returning just in time for me to wretch into the container. The burn of alcohol making its way back out of my mouth makes me feel like I am spitting flame. Kristen holds the basin for me, and then sets it on the floor as I return my head to the couch. I'm sweating profusely and can't seem too cool down no matter what I do. I feel a wet hand towel appear on my forehead as Kristen walks by and takes a seat on the chair next to me. She's making this as easy as she can for me. I greatly appreciate her every move.

My eyes are dry and difficult to keep open, the little bit of light visible in the room is enough to make my head pound out of control. Every muscle in my body aches like it has been pounded to mush with a sledgehammer. I can barely find the strength to roll over far enough to throw up in the basin. Kristen stands watch in case I need anything. The embarrassment washes over me whenever I realize this. I owe her so much.

Every hour I throw up about four times, even though there is nothing at all in my stomach. The dry heaving has gotten so violent that I can barely even do that anymore. The act of throwing up without any strength at all is a very odd sensation. It must be a pitiful sight to witness. I also experience periods of extreme coldness as well as violent sweats that make me feel like I have been set on fire. The shaking in my limbs has gotten slightly more stable, but I am still a prisoner to the couch due to the muscle fatigue. I have gone through three-quarters of the bottle of vodka by the time I finally start to feel some relief.

I don't know what time it is, or even what section of the day it is. The pain that followed the overdose has completely disoriented me. Kristen is in the chair asleep and its dark in the house still. I figure that it must be close to midnight. I look at the cable box to find that it reads 5:27am. Holy shit. I had no idea that it was already early morning. Kristen must not be going to work today; otherwise she would already be in the shower. I straighten up slowly and set my feet on the ground deciding to give standing a shot. I lift myself off of the couch for the first time in what seems like days, and manage to hold my own weight successfully. My body still feels like it has been through the war, but at least now I am actually able to function on my own. I walk out to the kitchen to find a bottle of water; it's the only thing that sounds good at the moment. Kristen wakes up right after me, and tells me that she is going to get ready for work and just go in a bit late. I nod sheepishly and make my way upstairs to get some actual sleep in her bed.

She gets ready quickly and sits on the foot of the bed waiting for me to acknowledge her. I look at her and notice that she has a few tears welled up in her eyes and an odd look on her face. I'm not sure what to say or do, so I tell her that I'm sorry. She cracks a small smile and lets a tear fall then whispers "No, I am."

I ask her what she's talking about, but she just slowly shakes her head and runs her hand down my shoulder. She leans in and gives me a kiss, then walks out of the bedroom. I hear her leave and fall back asleep, my head swimming in confusion.

36. Crush

As I suspected I'll be going to the little gathering tonight by myself. That's probably better anyway; Nikki only cares about herself lately. She'd most likely make a spectacle of herself, and just make everyone that much more uncomfortable. I don't understand what her problem is, but she's been really weird ever since she picked me up from rehab. It never used to be like this. We used to be a team. Both when we were clean together, and afterward when we weren't. Either way, she never treated me the way that she does now. It's as if I'm just an employee in the house. I love her to death however, which just makes it that much more painful. I have no idea what to do to make things better, so I'm just going to plod along as usual and hope that it's just the drugs talking.

I try to fight the sadness as I drive on the winding roads through the countryside. I can't believe the direction that my life has taken. I can't believe the consequences that I have had to see and endure due to what my life has become. I just saw this kid a week or so before I got picked up and tossed into rehab. The artsy little town that I am going to is only about ten miles away from my golden city of heroin. Incidentally, it's also where I get clean needles from the needle exchange they have setup. Because of the towns' close proximity to the source; you end up running into old friends on a regular basis. This kid was one of the friends that I saw all the time.

He was an amazing artist and kept to himself mostly. Never causing harm to anyone – just afflicted with a bad heroin addiction. He had a small studio apartment near downtown, and would hang out painting and working on new pieces whenever he had even a moment of free time. The thing that used to always blow me away was how talented he actually was. I have never witnessed anyone put their mind down on canvas as effectively as he could. He could use any medium his heart desired, as long as it pertained to the nature of the piece itself. Materials where never an obstacle, he always knew exactly what was needed to accomplish whatever he was working on. He was a genius beyond my comprehension, and now he's gone. Gone because of a drug. Gone because of my drug.

There are so many people in this world that will never bear witness to the amazing talents this kid was able to bring into the world. Even after his death, he'll just be seen as another junkie who got sucked into the drug game and ultimately screwed up to the point of death. That will be what society sees him as, and nothing more. That is what he will be remembered as – a good for nothing junkie. The only people who will know his true story will be his friends, because we are the only ones that have the ability to see past the drug use, and the lifestyle that goes with it. This makes me very angry and even sadder the more I think about it. At least we're all getting together for him tonight.

I pull into the usual parking lot which ends up costing me nothing because it's after 4:00pm. There's a litany of parking places to choose from, so I throw the truck in one of them and jump out. The park is a ten minute walk from here, so I'll be there in no time at all. Walking these familiar streets makes me think about Kristen, who I haven't spoken to in a few months now. Things have just gotten so out of control on my end, I'd rather not suck her into the madness. She knows this and has no resentment toward me. She wishes everyday that I would get the necessary help and kick the habit, but after failing so many times, I don't see that happening anytime soon. I wish I could update her from time to time just to let her know that I'm ok, but I can't do it yet. I know that she worries.

In the corner of the park by the tree line I see a small congregation of people that I recognize. I walk across the damp grass slowly fighting the lump in my throat that rises with each step I make closer to the huddle. All of the faces acknowledge my presence and a few hugs are given out. We are gathered around some lit candles, a picture of my friend, and some of his paintings that he especially liked. At some point during the vigil we all join hands in silence as I hear some sobbing from a girl that was in love with him right up until the very end.

He was found in his apartment face down on the floor with a brush in his hand and a piece of canvas on the easel in front of him with barely any paint on it. The estimation is that he was dead for three days before anybody found him. The girl that was just crying was actually the person who went looking for him and got very worried when he didn't answer his door. She called the police out of desperation and they gained access to his apartment. This is the story that another guy here was telling me after we decided to chill out for a little bit a few feet away from the small shrine.

There was some signal that I had apparently missed, but we were all about to get high. Someone had brought some dope and retreated to just inside the tree line to cook up. It seemed as though the pain was simply too much to bear without the help of our faithful substance. I was offered a needle, being told that it was fresh and clean as they had brought a small supply for anyone who had showed up. How could I decline? I couldn't. I gladly took it and retreated into the tree line out of sight to administer my medication.

I walked back toward the group feeling slightly more numb. The hit had helped, but it didn't relieve all the pain. Being here felt especially creepy, seeing his artwork right there in front of me, but knowing that he was gone forever was almost too much for me to take. I felt like I was going to have a mental breakdown, and couldn't figure out how to control myself. I can't do this here. Not in front of these people, it would just make everything so much harder for them as well. I quickly thanked everyone and made my way back to the parking lot. I couldn't take it anymore. I was reminded of my own situation too much while standing there. A wave of depression has started to wrap itself around me. I need to get out of here as quickly as I can, and I have a long drive back home still. I find my way back to the truck, dodging traffic appropriately so that I didn't get hit by some crazy person. Once inside I take a deep breath, realizing that I now have to drive under the influence, and on the brink of losing my mind completely. I pull out of the parking lot, being extra careful, and head to the long winding road back home.

On my way home all I can think about is how this is all going to end ultimately. I can't seem to tear myself away from the ugly truth that if I stay doing what I am doing – I am going to die. I can't seem to find a feasible plan that will keep me away from death, unless I stop using completely and manage to stay clean for more than eight hours. I need to get control of myself so that I don't end up like all of my friends who have taken things to the point of death. Nikki has got to get out of my life completely, or I fear that I will never ever even have a chance at changing. She is the most self-destructive person I know, and will never be able to help me stay clean in any way. Keeping myself away from her is going to be extremely hard, she's like another one of my addictions. I have no idea how to execute any of these thoughts, but at least I am having them, that's one step in the right direction I think.

Just then a small group of deer run right out into the road from the woods to my right. I slam on the breaks and the truck starts to skid out of control, clearly not able to stop at that rate of speed. I fumble at the wheel trying to avoid hitting any of the deer as they freeze in front of me on the road, not sure which way to run to avoid the out of control vehicle. I yank on the wheel one last time to the right and the truck turns sideways starting to veer off of the road. The front of the truck straightens out at the last instant and smashes into a large tree on the side of the road sending my head directly into the windshield.

37. Surprise

I am startled out of my sleep when I hear banging on the door. It's 8:05am according to the alarm clock on Kristen's nightstand. Who could possibly be here? I get up and throw on some clothes that I had on the floor next to the bed and make my way down the stairs. I open the door only to be greeted by three police officers with a couple of medics behind them. The one in front reads me my rights and explains that I have been sectioned by a family member.

I'm in a complete state of shock and awe. Not knowing what to make of all this new information I stand there frozen. The police move about me wearily until I can feel the cold steel of handcuffs around my wrists. I don't even know where they are going to be taking me, as far I know no crime has actually been committed. This is not my main concern however. My main concern is what family member knows about my addiction? What has happened? It's not until I am in the cruiser and on my way to the court house that I figure it all out.

Kristen told me that she was sorry this morning because she knew that she was going to call my mother and let her know what I've been up to. Last night scared her to that point, and I really can't blame her for doing it. This is really going to turn my world upside down. I don't even want to think about my protected family members seeing me in this way. I must look beyond disheveled. Fuck.

They haul me out of the back of the car and lead me into the rear of the courthouse. Trials are waiting to begin, and I am going to be waiting until what is already scheduled has completed. I'm ushered into the convict side of the court room, even though I have committed no crime. I try to keep my eyes forward for as long as I can before peering out into the audience section of the courtroom. My mother is there, crying silently.

Next to her are my grandparents, who I cannot even make eye contact with. Finally off to the right of them, staring at me with a blank look on his face – my brother. I notice that I'm wearing one of his shirts as I stand here cuffed amongst the other detained criminals. With a flick of a switch, one of my worst nightmares has come true.

Two hours later it's time for my little trial to begin. The judge calls my mother up to talk seeing as how she is the one who had me sectioned. She goes on to give a pretty accurate account of what happened to me last night as Kristen must have spared her no detail. The judge nods with an astute understanding, and sentences me to a mandatory two week stay at a local rehabilitation center. Another nightmare come true, how many more will there be? That appears to be the end of it, and the arresting police officers are kind enough to let me have ten minutes with my family before trucking me off to hell. Honestly I don't know which is worse at this point, facing them or facing sobriety.

One by one they hug me, not saying a word. My mother is crying profusely but doing her best to keep it together. Having just learned about my addiction a few hours ago – I give her a lot of credit. My grandparents are also doing a good job at not showing their immense disappointment in me, but I know that it's there. My brother gives me a look of utter confusion and tells me to get better. The next thing I know I'm being dropped off in front of a local hospital that has a rehab center conveniently attached to it. I have no idea how I am going to get through this, especially after last night. I haven't even been able to use once since then, which leaves me with just my last experience – the horrible overdose itself. That really sucks. Now I'm supposed to walk into this place and magically come out the other end a changed person and clean as a whistle. Even after the close brush with death of last night, all I can think about is stuffing my veins with heroin. This is going to be anything but easy.

Surprise

I learn quickly that the structure in place here is less than desirable, but I have no choice so I decide not to fight it. The staff members all seem really nice, but in a fake sort of way, and I can't really put my finger on the specific traits that leave a cheap taste in my mouth. The other people that are here seeking help seem to be in far worse shape than I am. The stories that get told are sometimes eye openers even for me, but I'll never let things get to that point. They have me on a regimen of drugs that helped immensely with the detox, and continue to keep me on an even keel, even though the drug itself has all but left my system. The mental addiction is still as strong as it was when I first walked into this place.

Everything seemed to be going normal until about the 4th day in. I was keeping busy and really felt as though I could overcome this terrible drug, as long as I kept my mind occupied and away from it completely. I needed to disassociate with people that were involved with it and still used, which I pretty much have already accomplished for the most part. I'm filled with a powerful feeling of hope, that somehow I'll be able to make this all work again and reclaim my life. Perhaps this time I'll get a real job and not become some robot at a fucking grocery store. I'm sure that fixing things like that will really help toward keeping me on track. Yes, things seemed to have been going very well – and then I saw her.

She was a new arrival. She must have shown up yesterday at the earliest, otherwise I would have already noticed her. Long straight black hair and thin as a rail. She was beautiful. I had to talk to her. I was drawn to her in the same manner that I was drawn to heroin. No control at all over my actions, I walked right up to her and asked her what her name was.

"Nikki" she replied.

That was it. Just hearing the sound of her voice made me weak. I had to find a way to get her alone, even if the rules here are extremely strict about male/female relations. I had to. I didn't have a choice, and it appeared as though she shared some of the same feelings as I. Amazing.

We found a table in the common area and started getting to know each other. She was here on her own accord fighting a cocaine addiction. She wanted to get clean and have some good ammo behind her at her next hearing for custody. She was married for a short time and has a four year old son that she is not allowed to see unsupervised due to her drug addiction. Her ex-husband currently has custody and is adamant that she stays away from him as much as possible, unless she is actually clean. I couldn't even imagine her using a drug, her face seemed so innocent. I suppose that I was blinded by my own feelings toward her, which in themselves are still quite unexplainable.

Later on that night I found a way to sneak out of my room and meet her in a janitor's closet that for some reason doesn't seem to get much use. Once inside we didn't even have to speak one word, clothes started to find their way to the floor. We fucked for what seemed like hours, both enjoying ourselves beyond comprehension. It was exactly what I needed. We were able to get out of the closet and back into our rooms without being caught. This was certainly going to make the rest of my stay here far more interesting. I went to sleep that night thanking my "higher power" for bringing me to this place. I almost didn't even have the opportunity to meet her.

38. Lucky

Red and blue lights fill my blurred vision. Tiny pieces of glass fall off of my head and down my face as I pull back from the smashed windshield. I can feel the wetness from the blood on my forehead, I'm afraid to move or touch my face not knowing the full extent of the damage. My head is pounding like twelve boxers are all taking turns using it as a training bag. Nothing else on my body seems to be affected or broken. I sit still in the seat waiting for someone to come.

An ambulance pulls in next to the truck and paramedics rush to my door. I hear the commotion of muffled voices and radios going off all around me, the flashing lights put me into a trance. My door is opened and people are frantically checking me out to make sure that I'm alive and not in a mangled condition. Carefully I'm removed from the truck.

I can hear the paramedics fighting with the police officers who are insisting on giving me a breathalyzer test as they hoist me onto a stretcher. They strap a neck brace around me just to be safe, and load me into an ambulance. The paramedics tell the police that they smell no sign of alcohol on my breath and that they need to get me to a hospital. Reluctantly they leave, and we begin the long journey.

"Deer" I say to the guys in the back with me.

They nod their heads in understanding, and tell me to just relax. There's a thought. Just relax. How? How could I possibly just relax? My life is falling apart all over again, just in different ways than before. That's always how it happens though, I get one thing wrapped up and another completely falls apart. I definitely cannot win.

With the heroin still making its way through my system, I feel no pain at all. My arm could be lopped off at the elbow and I'm sure that I wouldn't even feel it. This is both good and bad.

Good because I am perfectly comfortable, bad because I don't know the extent of the injuries, and I really don't want to. The neck brace is an especially nice touch, making it basically impossible for me to move. It's like I have been locked into an extra firm pillow. It sounds like it should be comfortable, but it's not at all. I can't wait for them to take it off.

We make it to the emergency room and they wheel me inside with a sense of urgency. Once inside I'm swarmed with doctors all poking and prodding trying to rule out any invisible dangers such as internal bleeding. As it all turns out there is nothing wrong with me at all except for some cuts and scrapes on my forehead from the windshield. I apparently smacked it just right, sustaining only a mild concussion from the blow. They decide to keep me here overnight just for my own comfort and tell me that I should be all set to leave in the morning.

Nikki is going to be pissed about the truck, but honestly it didn't look that bad from what I saw of it. Who knows though, I'm no mechanic, it could be totally wrecked. Part of me doesn't even care – let her be mad, she'll get over it eventually. I drift off to sleep and enjoy the pain meds that they didn't need to give me.

Morning comes and the nurse tells me I can leave. I get out of the hospital bed and put on my clothes from last night. Rather than dealing with any other bullshit I decide to call my brother to come get me. He tells me he'll be there in twenty minutes and waiting by the front door. When I walk out he's the first car I see. I slowly climb in the passenger side and light up a smoke.

"What the fuck happened to you?" He asks.

"I hit a tree last night trying to avoid a bunch of deer in the road...I just got a concussion though, it's all good." I reply as carelessly as I can.

We decide to take a quick ride before he brings me back to my place. I lie and tell him that I'm clean when he asks. I don't like doing that, but it is my ultimate goal – to get clean and stay that way. So it only feels like a half lie. I can tell that he probably has his own theories anyways, but he spares me of the details, which is nice. We stop at a gas station to get some coffee and head back to my place. Once inside I see no sign of Nikki. She must have actually gone to work, which is shocking to me. Not to mention that she most likely has no idea what happened to me last night, or the truck for that matter. She probably figures that I crashed at someone's house last night, not knowing that I actually crashed into a tree instead.

My brother and I take a seat on the couch and light up a joint for old time's sake, this time he brought one over and hooked me up. He tells me about some of the courses he's taking in college – substance abuse is one of them, we both laugh. I don't know how he manages to work full time, go to school and still find time to get high and have fun. He's five years younger than me and already has a much better plan in place for dealing with life than I ever did. I find myself being jealous of these qualities, as I wish that I could possess them, even just a few of them. Anything at this point would be helpful. I obviously can't seem to get anything right. Not even 24 hours pass from one disaster to another anymore. I just need to be locked in a room somewhere and constantly monitored by someone that has an entire brain in their head. I shudder at that thought as I realize I just described prison. I really am a mess.

Just then my brother's cell phone rings and he answers it with a strange look on his face. He looks at me and holds the phone out.

"It's for you."

The grocery store has called back and wants me to come in for an interview tomorrow at 11:00am. Wow, that was easy enough. They told me that they think they have a position stocking shelves and just need to go over some basics in the morning. I better look my best; hopefully the horrific scratches on my head clear up a little by morning. My brother is very happy that I'm so close to getting another job. He's very supportive considering it is just a job at a grocery store stocking shelves. His enthusiasm seems very genuine though. In some ways I think he's happier about it than I am. He pulls out another joint and looks at me.

"Let's celebrate."

He doesn't have to tell me twice. I take a big pull and sink deeper into the couch trying to relax my throbbing head. It still hurts like hell, but slightly less than it did last night when I arrived at the hospital. I vaguely explain to my brother where I was last night. He asks if I used, to which I reply no – again. That's the one thing that really sucks about being an addict. Nobody ever takes your word for anything, then again, they know better. He knows that I used – no matter how many times I say "no I didn't" or "I've been clean" he knows that I didn't get out of there last night without using. He also knows that me being high probably didn't help my attempt at avoiding that tree on the side of the road. Regardless I stand my ground and insist that I was clean, just to avoid the conversation, sometimes I can be such a coward.

My brother announces that he has to go back to the school to make his last class. I say goodbye and retreat to the bedroom. Plopping myself down on the bed I bury myself in blankets and hope that my head will stop throbbing soon.

39. Freedom

The rest of my stay here at rehab villa went really fast, due to my new companion. Nikki and I had clearly become a "thing", and everyone knew it. Relationships in rehab are frowned upon, therefore we tried to keep things as inconspicuous as possible, but that was very hard to do. I got caught in her bed one night when her roommate finally got sick of lying for us. At least I had found the one thing that was able to keep my mind off of heroin - for the most part. I only had one more day to go, and she was getting out the following day. We set it all up so that she would come and pick me up at my mother's house the day she got out. We would then stay at her parent's house a few towns over and a few towns closer to my favorite city. We both had every intention of staying clean from that point out. At least that was our plan.

The day finally came – it was time to leave. I was going to face my family for the first time since the courthouse drama two weeks ago. This should be interesting. I had been talking to my mother on the phone every couple of days while I was in here, filling her in briefly on the events that helped to lead up to this. She was oblivious and it took her a long time to adjust to the new information. She had been relaying things to my grandparents and ultimately to my brother. He'd be the only one at the house tonight when I got there. Evan was coming to pick me up from rehab; he wanted to see how I was handling things anyways. He was late which irritated me, but he showed up eventually and we got the fuck out of there.

The whole ride up to the house I talked to him all about Nikki. He seemed skeptical of my sudden love interest, but supportive nonetheless. Either way I'll be glad to get rid of this place when she does get out, a change of scenery will definitely do me good. Evan drives me up to my house and I hop out and go inside.

I haven't been here in months and it all seems so different. My brother has not yet taken over the room that we shared for so many years. My side is still completely intact only missing what I took to Dave's with me - the essentials really. My brother had already made arrangements with a friend of his and retrieved my car from Kristen's a day or so after I went into rehab, so that was here waiting for me as well. When Nikki gets out she's going to meet me here and then we will drive in tandem to her parent's house. My brother knows nothing of Nikki yet.

My brother leads me outside to share a joint with me, and I tell him some of the highlights of rehab. Like the scavengers hunt that they had as a special New Years activity. I won a coffee mug that night filled with chocolates and a small stuffed white bear. That was the only prize I won during my two week stay. That was it – no gold stars, no cute little pens with logos on them, nothing else. I guess I'm good at scavenger hunts. Who knew?

I then lead right into the topic of Nikki, telling my brother all about her and really talking her up. I can see the skepticism in his eyes as well. For some reason everybody thinks that this isn't a good idea, they don't tell my why necessarily, but I can tell that they are apprehensive about it. Maybe because it was so soon. Maybe because we met in rehab. Maybe because I'm insane and talk like a crazy person. I can't rule out any of these possibilities.

I tell my brother that she's coming to get me tomorrow when she gets out and then we're going to hit the road and shack up at her parent's house for a little bit.

"You're only going to sleep here tonight?" He asks with a bewildered tone.

"Yeah, I don't ever sleep here so what's the big deal?" I ask back.

"I just thought that you'd be taking it easy for a little while that's all."

I don't need to "take it easy". That's such a weird concept. Should I just sit around all day not doing anything because I might use if I do? That doesn't make any sense to me at all. I don't understand all of the concern, and I certainly don't understand why suddenly I'm this fragile little thing that needs to be talked to like I'm twelve. I overdosed – once. It's over. I just want to get on with things now. I just want to actually seek out some happiness in the world, and I don't understand why that is such a bad thing. It's ok for me to get completely brainwashed for two weeks in an institution, but it's not ok for me to try to get on with my life afterward. I don't get it.

I explain to my brother that I'm fine and have finally found someone that really makes me feel good about myself. He still seems a bit apprehensive, but I'm sure he'll understand once he meets her. My mother will be home shortly, I'm sure that I'll be up for awhile tonight talking to her. I'm not really sure what to tell her about the heroin, it's not exactly a subject that I'm comfortable talking to anyone about. I'll just have to see how things go when she gets here. I know it's not going to be long before my brother's curious little mind gets the best of him and he'll be asking me all sorts of questions about my addiction.

I notice that I'm still wearing my hospital bracelet, so I run over to the silverware drawer and cut if off with a knife. I then reach over and place it on the fridge. Just like displaying an "A" paper. Why not? It's certainly the best accomplishment that I've had in years. I'm officially jobless at the moment, as I called up the wonderful little grocery store that I work at from within rehab to offer an explanation for my disappearance and was informed that they had already terminated me. Nice. There's something about being told you were terminated that sounds so violent. Whatever, I hated it there anyway, maybe being terminated could end up being a good thing.

My mother arrived and we both took a seat at the kitchen table realizing that it was going to be a long night. My brother was going out with some of his friends so nobody else would be here except for my step father. We talked for a few hours and I tried to comfort my mother by letting her know that she didn't do anything wrong that lead me to heroin use. This was by far one of her biggest concerns. She felt as though her parenting had somehow led me off course and right into the hands of drugs. This couldn't be farther from the truth. I knew full well what I was doing when I decided to take that needle from Brad the night he introduced me to the wonderful mixture. And I couldn't deny the way that it made me feel. The way it made me feel complete, and able to deal with anything that came my way. The way that it made me feel as though I had a purpose here amongst the brain dead crowd I'm always surrounded by. I do my best to ease her mind on all of the points that she brings up, but it still doesn't seem to make her less sad in the long run.

40. Interview

After a long sleep I begin to prepare myself for the interview at the grocery store a few blocks away. Nikki is in the bathroom illustrating her latest addiction – bulimia. I figured it all out last night when she was promptly sick as soon as she stepped foot in the door. I didn't know at the time, but found out later that she had just eaten her free meal at the restaurant she works at. She was also obsessing about her weight all night standing in front of the mirror for long periods of time. Nikki is about 5'4 and weighs approximately 110 pounds. There's not an ounce of fat on her entire body, yet suddenly she thinks that she should be on a diet. Just like anything else – Nikki has managed to get herself completely engrossed with the idea of throwing up after she eats anything that resembles food.

I've decided to not entertain her new "affliction", and do everything I can to not call attention to it. She's going to end up in rough shape at some point. Between the drug use and now the incessant puking, I predict that she'll be in the hospital by next week sometime. She has completely spiraled out of control ever since we fucked shit up at her parent's house and ended up living in the truck for two months. Now we have this apartment, which was handed to us, and she's just going to throw it all away. She's not even going to try, that's what pisses me off the most. I at least like to think that, for the most part, I put in some effort before burning my whole world down. A small little minuscule amount of effort at least. She does not. She lets it all go to shit right away without even thinking twice about preventing the impending disaster. It's like she doesn't realize that consequences for her actions actually exist. She doesn't take into account how one action might affect another, and ultimately what that will look like in the end. This is why she's always trying to find a way to beat the system, because she is emphatically incapable of following it – ever.

I put on the best clothes that I can find and hope that they are sufficient enough for an interview at a grocery store. I grab the key to the apartment and head to the street. The truck has been towed to a local garage around the corner from where I smashed into the tree. There's an insurance deductible involved in getting the claim money due to me being the person at fault for the accident. Last I checked deer didn't carry insurance cards on them. Nikki's parents are picking up the deductible cost, naturally, so the truck should be back in about a week or so. For now I'm on foot back and forth to my new job, if I get hired that is – at least it's close. I will need to find some sort of transportation down to the magical city soon, as our supply is getting somewhat low. That's going to turn into a problem soon, so I'd rather take care of it as quickly as I can.

I walk into the grocery store and once again make my way to the service desk. The same cute little girl is there working the counter, flashing her straight, white teeth at me – makes me think of Kristen. I tell her my name and that I'm here to see the manager for an interview. She smiles even wider and tells me to wait right there – she'll go get him. I turn around and evaluate my potential co-workers lined up on the front end. Mostly older housewives with a few younger people mixed in here and there. These are the kids that don't have rich parents. These are the kids that don't have the privilege of attending a $40,000 dollar per year University. These are the kids that I usually don't have a problem talking to. I then remember that I won't really see many of these people anyways as I'll be in the background stocking shelves all by myself. The sound of that alone is already very soothing in my head.

The manager comes around from behind the desk and shakes my hand while introducing himself – Jim something. We walk upstairs together and he makes small talk just like any other normal consumer. Once we get there he tells me to have a seat in the conference room and that he'll be right in. I sit in one of the metal framed chairs equipped with the black vinyl pad that's made just for your ass. I already can't wait to stand back up again.

Jim comes back in carrying a thin folder full of papers, and a couple of pens. His name tag affixed to his cheap button down stripped shirt is gleaming proudly, and couldn't look more out of place. I still don't register what his last name is. He hands me a pen and tosses the first sheet of paper at me explaining that it's a safety waiver of some sort which I need to sign. Then the next paper comes – another waiver. A waiver explaining that I have watched the sexual harassment video. A waiver for the loss prevention video. A waiver for the blood borne pathogen video. I sign them all, one by one. Jim explains that this is how they save time, and that I can skip out on two hours of terribly constructed instructional videos. I'm all for it. Jim's not so bad after all with his crazy eyes and sporadically grown beard.

He tells me that I'll be hired at minimum wage plus one dollar on top of that per hour. Sounds like a strange little system, but once again – I'm all for it. If someone is going to pay me to put boxes on a shelf over and over again – I'm all for it. I didn't realize that I was already hired when I walked in the door this morning, so that's also very cool. I didn't even have to sit here and talk a bunch of bullshit trying to get this meaningless job. The less work that I have to do to, the better – I'm all for it.

Jim takes me on short little tour throughout the store, showing me the back room where I'll be working out of all night. I do my best to remember some of the names that he tells me so that I can come in and meet my boss later this week on my first day. I have two days to rest up until then. My first night will be a 6:00pm-midnight shift, and my supervisor will only be here until 8:00pm that night. So I'll get acquainted with him quickly and then I'm on my own until midnight. It sounds great to me, and I can't wait to actually start making money while acting like a robot. I don't think that I am going to dread going to work nearly as much as I used to when I was dealing with the "numbers" all night long. I swear that job almost actually took my life at times. It certainly sucked the life right out of me from the minute I stepped foot in the door at the beginning of every shift. I'm glad to be rid of it.

I walk back to the apartment feeling good about myself. I actually have employment again; something that I never thought would even happen. I know that it's a bullshit job at a grocery store, but at least I'm not some homeless bum earning money by ripping off stores. Perhaps I can even keep my mind off of the heroin a little. Although right now it's calling to me from blocks away. Nikki will either be at work or in a coma by the time that I get there, which means I'll have the entire house to myself either way. I can't wait to get high. I can't wait to feel the rush again. I can't wait to make the world disappear.

41. Persuasion

Nikki finds the house without any problems, and within ten minutes of her arrival we are off, driving through the woods thirty miles away from her parent's house. I'm excited to be on this little adventure. I know that it has all happened very quickly, but it all seems so natural. Not to mention the fact that I can't stop thinking about her day and night. Nikki told me that her room was gigantic and that she has already talked to her parents about me coming to stay. Apparently they have no problem with it. I find this as a little odd, but decide to go with it – one less obstacle in the way of our happiness.

We finally arrive at the foot of a long windy dirt driveway that climbs high atop a small mountain. The house is very large from the outside and delicately ornate. A long porch starts at the front and wraps around both sides of the house. You could play baseball on the porch alone it's so large. I'm not used to places like this. Nikki drags me up the front steps and opens the door with her free hand, which I notice is unlocked. Another thing I'm not very used to. I guess there's no need to lock your doors if you live in the middle of the woods with nobody around you for miles. It still just feels wrong for some reason.

Her parents are hanging out in the living room not paying much attention to the TV that is on in the background. Her father is reading some sort of book which he glances up from with a big toothy grin. I immediately think that he's a little odd. Her mother is thumbing through a magazine and sipping on some sort of fruity drink. She must be the alcoholic in the family. They both act as if they have already met me, and that they love me. Nikki and I scurry up to her room to get rid of the bags of clothes that I brought from my house. Her room is gigantic – exactly as she described – wood floors throughout and a tall peaked ceiling adorned with two elaborate ceiling fans. She has her own queen sized bed which I immediately think will be a lot of fun. Other than that her room is somewhat bare. I like it. The windows are very large, and go all the way to the floor – also very cool. Of course there's not really any kind of view to be seen except for trees, but still I find it soothing. It's certainly a big change from the little tiny room that I'm used to sharing with my brother back home. This is going to be a lot of fun, and her parents seem whacky enough that they won't get in the way at all.

I look over at Nikki just in time to see her ladle some white powder out of a small baggie with her finger and shove it into her nostril.

"What are you doing?" I yell in my best whisper.

"It's just some extra shit I had stashed." She explains as she tosses me the baggie.

I've never been a very big fan of coke, but I'm not above doing it. I don't understand why she is already using again after just getting out of rehab this morning. I reach in reluctantly with my finger and get just enough to catch a buzz. Nikki comes running over to me tearing off her top in the process. She wraps her arms around me and drags me over to the bed; I drop the baggie on the floor. She starts to claw her way through my clothing until I am wearing nothing at all – I do the same to her. The heat from her body is radiating all around her, melting my thoughts and causing me to act out of pure instinct.

I wind my way around her so that we are fit together perfectly like two puzzle pieces. My hands moving a mile a minute but slow enough to enjoy every perfect curve and divot of her body. This continues until I simply can't stand it anymore. Until I have to be inside of her before I die from sheer frustration. I climb up on top of her and find her perfect center. It's waiting for me patiently, and ready for whatever comes its way. My mind is off completely. I'm all consumed by the power of our bodies together, and am completely dedicated to our movements. The physical sensations are indescribable and very close to the rush I feel when using. Entirely different sensations, but ultimately on the same level as shooting my most favorite strain of heroin. Things come to fruition, on their own, after what seems like a decade of time. I could do that all day long.

Nikki starts asking me about heroin while we are lying in bed together. She wants to know what it feels like. She says that she has never done it, but always wanted to, and is very curious as to how it differs from the drugs that she is already acquainted with. I try to explain to her the best I can, but ultimately tell her that there really isn't a good way to describe it without feeling it firsthand. She immediately wants to go get some. I tell her no. I tell her that I really need to stay away from it, and how badly it screwed up my life. I tell her all about the overdosing episode at Kristen's house which was what landed me in rehab to begin with. I tell her what happened to Brad that night when I found him face down on the floor all fucked up and close to death. I tell her about the constant pull it has on your mind no matter what you are doing. I even tell her about the dangers of copping the shit out in the magical city fifteen miles away from here.

She still wants to try it. She still wants to feel it for herself. She still wants to know why everyone who is addicted to heroin loves it so much. She wants an addiction to mean that much to her. She wants it bad enough that she'll even aid in facilitating my own relapse. I've fallen in love with the devil. Again. The first time was with heroin itself. And now I'm really not going to be able to get away from it. It's as if the heroin gods have sent Nikki here to pull me back in by whatever means necessary. Like I needed another hook. I have no idea what to do as I am faced with this enormous conflict within me. It would be really fun to use with someone like Nikki, and of course that fact alone doesn't help my cravings. I tell her that I at least need the night to think about it and that we aren't going anywhere right now.

She seems unsatisfied with my decision, but pulls the little baggie of coke back out and takes another hit. I'm starting to surmise that Nikki didn't go to rehab with any real intentions of getting clean. She did it as a show for the courts. She is trying to prove that she is a fit mother and has no drug dependencies of any kind. Her parents are helping with the facade by giving her a wonderful place to live and a seemingly endless supply of cash as needed. Not to mention the fact that they conveniently never ask her any questions. In their eyes, Nikki can do no wrong. This is going to get completely out of control. I can feel it.

42.   First Night

ikki walks into the apartment three hours earlier than
her shift was supposed to end at the restaurant.. I know
instantly that there is a problem. She has been stealing
money from the register. Daily. They finally caught on after
about two weeks of her continuous behavior. Of course they
can't prove anything except for what happened today, because
somebody actually saw her do it. She was performing this little
act at the same time everyday, which was the only time that she
was left as the sole employee in the building. The manager goes
outside for her 2:00pm smoke break everyday – and right on
time. This is also during a shift change that leaves the two of
them the only employees there on most days. It's just the way
that it works out. After the manager suspected Nikki of stealing
from the register, she decided to pinpoint when exactly she was
getting away with it. So today she decided to pretend that she
was going out for her regularly scheduled smoke break, but
instead kept an eye on the register from behind a separation wall
by the kitchen entrance. Within two minutes Nikki had already
pocketed her take for the day from the register and was caught
red handed. That was the end of her waitressing career.

So here she is - unemployed, puking every few hours due
to her latest obsession with bulimia, and fighting withdrawal all
the time by shooting up whenever she gets a chance. Luckily I
have a job, but with the shit pay that I'll make every week we'll
get nowhere fast. Nikki is obviously going to be incapable of
holding a job for more than a week before committing a crime. I
really have no idea how to get out of this mess – unless it's
without her. I can't even bear to think about what that would be
like though. I can't be without her. She's another one of my
addictions.

She's pissed off that she got caught, as she always is when something like this happens. She always acts like she wasn't doing anything wrong, and appalled by the possibility of consequences for her actions. I know that she's like this, yet it still surprises me every time something like this happens. I have no idea why I am still capable of shock when it comes to her. I haven't been with her physically since a few weeks after we got out of rehab; I think that the heroin has taken away our sex drive. This is a real downer, because sex is one of the things that always glued us together – we have the ability to drive each other completely out of control. I suppose that a relationship should be based on much more than just the physical attraction, but we definitely have most of our strengths there. Still I can't manage to leave her, or even really consider the option. No matter how fucked up everything gets – she's still really the only person that I have in my corner.

She sees me looking at her, and immediately goes to the bedroom to look for a needle and some fresh brown powder. I knew that she'd run right to it, especially now that she has the job excuse to be upset with. I continue to chill out, preparing myself for my first night of work in months at the grocery store down the road. I'm going to do whatever I can to not let her get me down. I also don't want to use before going to work on my first day. So I try to keep things nice and relaxing. I can get high when I get home at 12:30pm tonight. I can make it until then.

I still have to figure out transportation for the next couple of days so that I can make the trip down to drug land and score some more dope. I think that I'll give Evan a call later and see if he'll let me borrow his car, I'm sure he'll agree to it. I'll just have to make it lucrative for him somehow. I'll call him from the payphone at work on my first break.

I get to work and meet my new boss, his name is Tom. He's a normal blue color guy that pretty much does the same thing every day of his life. I managed to hear about his snowmobile collection and his favorite truck during the first fifteen minutes of my shift. Some people find comfort in just being an open book for the entire world to read. I will never understand this concept. Why he thinks that I give a shit about his snowmobiles is beyond me. I don't look like I ride snowmobiles. I don't even think I look like someone who knows what one is. That might be irrelevant though. Perhaps people like this just need someone to talk to about their useless pleasures. Perhaps they just want to tell everyone exactly who they are and what they like, as if making your motives more clear will translate into others liking you. I still don't get it.

My job consists of monitoring a predetermined set of items that change each week along with the sales flyer. I also will be keeping an eye on what is commonly referred to as the "staples" or the items that people buy no matter what is on sale. Those are basically my only tasks while I am here, unless the people that worked before me have some sort of special project that bleeds over into my shift. This is exactly the kind of job that I was looking for. A position that doesn't really ask too much of me, and keeps me away from constant interaction with anyone, especially the general public. I just zone right out into my own little world when I am around them. I don't understand any of the things that they say or do, and in turn it makes me feel like I'm losing my mind completely. This is perfect.

My first break comes and I run outside to smoke my lungs out of my chest and give Evan a call. I ask him if I can borrow the car, he agrees, but under one condition – that I use with him. He wants to know what it feels like. Fuck me. I've been down this road before. I tell him that I have to think about it, and that I don't like the idea at all. He tries to reassure me by telling me that he just wants to experiment, and that he's done everything else before, just not heroin. I hang up the phone with trembling fingers. I was not expecting this at all, especially from Evan.

I walk back into the store all consumed by this new crossroads. It makes my head burn like a migraine as the lights in the store suddenly seem like the brightest things on the planet. I don't know how to deal with this new problem. I have to really sit Evan down and explain to him that this is a onetime deal. I am not going to help him get shit in the future, or make using any easier for him. He gets a taste and then he walks – that's it. Unlike Brad, I am not looking for someone to keep me company while I get high all day long. I've already created the monster that I live with, and I'm not ruining anyone else's life. I refuse to do it. Not to mention the fact that Evan is a smart guy and knows the kind of shit heroin has gotten me into. I guess it never really bothered him as much as it should have, which explains why he's still around. Everyone else has all but faded away.

I wrap up the shift which seems to end in record time – nothing like working that fucking register. I'm sure stressing out about introducing Evan to the devil herself also made the time go by rather quickly. I walk out into the cold air and start making my way back home. I have tomorrow off so that would be the best time to grab Evan's car and hit the road. I am going to also make sure that he doesn't come with me, fuck that. Nikki has some kind of stash of cash somewhere that I need to get from her in order to cop some more shit. I don't expect a hassle from her as she'll be just as enthused about scoring the dope as I am - possibly even more.

So fuck it – I'll let Evan get high, under my supervision, and after he agrees to my rules.

43. Relocation

Nikki and I are on our way to the city early the next morning to score some dope. It's been a few weeks since I have been here. Eerily it all comes back to me in an instant. Even the air in the streets is exactly the same as I left it the last time I came down here to cop. My heart starts racing as I pull up to the old abandoned building – which is still completely unchanged on the outside. I walk past the begging junkies and stinking cats all the way to the center, to find that nobody is there. The door is open and nothing is inside except for a chair and some empty wooden shelves. How can this be? The place must have gotten raided. Goddammit. Now I actually have to talk to one of these fucking bums who are lying in the cat piss on the floor. I can still hear the dripping from one of the leaky water pipes that runs down the length of the hallway. I can't believe that I need to go to a new spot.

Like any good business man, however, the dealer had one of his worker bees standing by the exit door letting all of the usual customers know where the new location was. I guess I won't have to deal with a smelly junkie bum after all. Things are starting to look up. I get my instructions discreetly from the flunky while we hide in the shadows of the doorway. I'm on my way to a broken down house in a slightly rougher neighborhood deeper into the outskirts of the city lines. I'm a little nervous as I approach the house, and remember to park up the street a little bit so that it doesn't look too conspicuous. Out on foot I make my way up the path which leads to the door. Same setup as before but, now it's a bit more out in the open. I make the usual exchange and I'm on my way back to the car, eyes over my shoulders at all times. I'm starting to get really good at scoring, which is ironic if you think about it. I shouldn't even be here.

Nikki is sitting patiently in the truck waiting for me to get back. She's a little nervous but not nearly as much as I thought she would be. It turns out that Nikki is one tough little cookie. She even offered to go get the shit herself when she realized that we had to change locations. I told her no and closed the discussion completely. That was the end of it. I get us out of the neighborhood and back on track to her parent's house. I can tell that the close proximity of the city is also going to make it very hard not to visit. I'd be lying if I didn't say that the excitement has already filled my veins with fire as we drive home. I am really looking forward to the taste of my old friend. I am not looking forward to introducing it to Nikki, however, I am in fear of her addictive personality. I am afraid of how she is going to react to its wonderful indescribable effects. She is going to latch right onto it as I did. It's going to fill the same void within her as it did me. I know it. This is not going to end well.

We pull into her driveway and she all but jumps out of the passenger seat running into the house with me trailing behind. I wonder if she gets this excited every time before trying a new drug. I'm starting to find it all a bit amusing actually. Fuck it, I'm going to stop stressing about it and just try to have a good time. She knows what she is getting herself into; at least she is educated on the drug itself and realizes that it's highly addictive. I shouldn't be doing it, but that's beside the point, it has been way too fucking long, I deserve a hit. I start to sprint up the stairs to her bedroom hot on her heels.

I have the wooden box buried deep in one of the bags that I brought up to her room. Everything necessary is still in that box, waiting to be used. The little metal caps are spinning around inside like tops given to a little boy at Christmas. The needles are marching along to the beat of the wooden matches on the inside walls of the box. My veins are pulsing with each step that brings me closer to getting high. Nikki can have her shot, but not before I get mine.

Relocation

The initial rush hits me like it did the very first time, it's almost as if I took too much, but it stabilizes quickly and I know that I'm safe.

"That's some really good shit." I tell Nikki with enthusiasm. This packet had a little red skull stamped on the outside of it. A new strain. I can already feel the subtle differences flowing through me. I like it. It rivals the scorpion.

I make sure that Nikki's dose is even less than mine. She's not going to need much to feel the effects of this monster. I suck up her elixir and instruct her to make a fist. Sticking the needle carefully into her vein, I draw back some blood as usual, and send her on the most amazing ride of her life for the very first time. Her eyes widen ever so slightly as the tainted liquid starts racing through her system. She lets out a small sigh and smiles widely at me as if she was ten years old and I just handed her a three-layer cake specially made just for her. She hasn't even fully embarked on her journey and already she understands its draw. She now understands all of the motives behind every user there is. It all comes down to this feeling right here.

I watch her enjoy her first hit for hours. For some reason I like seeing her reactions to the drug being that this is her first time. It makes me think back to that first fateful night with Brad. I had no idea what I was walking into until he pulled out the needle and set me up with a hit. I was not disappointed at all. I see her going through all of the same revelations that I did. I see her opening her eyes at times amazed at the incredible feelings that she didn't realize existed before. I see her thinking new thoughts for the very first time, and I marvel at her beauty as she does so. I am also going through my own beautiful reunion with this wonderful drug. My thoughts are wrapped up in hers and the cyclone of stimulation is enough to make my head inflate like a balloon. All I want to do is take her in my arms, and spend the rest of eternity locked in this moment. I want this to be all there is in the world. Her with me, and the catalyst known as heroin will fill in all of the gaps from the absence of everything else.

I fall asleep staring at the ceiling fan swirling above me. I could focus on just one blade of the fan and watch it twirling against the contrast of the dark wooden rafters that it hangs from. The sound of the swishing blade was the most soothing noise that I had ever heard. I couldn't hear anything else in the house, just that one blade consistently rotating without ever skipping a beat. Nikki had already passed out, not being able to withstand the powerful heroin, as I sat there reveling in the magnificence of the ceiling fan. I had no thoughts at all. My mind was a blank easel being manipulated by the robotic appliance that hung above me. I stared for as long as I could and eventually gave in to its serenity.

44.   Evan

After having a long talk with Evan, I am now cruising down the highway on my way to cop. I am going to come pick him up when I get done, and he's going to stay at my place tonight with Nikki and me. He can't wait to see what it feels like to shoot up, but he isn't acting like Nikki did before her first time. I still don't like it at all, and think that it's a really horrendous idea, but I can only warn so much before that person ultimately makes their own decision. I am holding onto every thread of hope in my mind that he'll try it and move on, and not get sucked in by its ultimate power. I will try to do everything that I can to keep him away from it if need be. I hate being put into this position.

The day itself is dark and wet, which I'm happy about. Some people get all upset when it isn't sunny out, and personally I like the contrast. I like the feeling of sanctuary that can be found in the shadows or the small areas of darkness that are created by the clouds. I can do without the sun blaring in my face every single day. Overcast days are gorgeous in their own unique way.

Nikki was still glued to the bed this morning when Evan came and picked me up. She is running herself into the ground with her current behavior. Her health is rapidly fading and it's really starting to concern me. Every time I try to talk to her about it though – she won't listen to me. She gets angry and irate. She throws things in my general direction in small fits of rage. The little amount of dishes that we did have are all chipped and broken from her hurling them across the room at me. This is not Nikki. Correction: this is Nikki now, controlled by drugs and psychological eating disorders. She is going to need to be hospitalized if she doesn't wake up and get control of herself soon. I just hope that she does something before it's too late.

I've decided to park the car at a small shopping center about 5 blocks away from the old beat up house. I'm being extra careful today, down here all alone, and having been away for so long. I don't want to look awkward or new here. I don't want a vehicle associated with my presence either. Cars can be misunderstood and tend to make people look more suspicious. I need this to be quick, easy, and clean. No bullshit.

I park Evan's car and pocket the little key-fob after I set its alarm. That would have been handy back in the day. Perhaps an alarm could have prevented all of the tires on the truck from getting slashed. In truth it probably wouldn't even had made a difference. Off on foot down the familiar street toward the house, I can smell those stale scents in the air. The car pollution smell that never seems to go away, no matter what time of the day it is. The food smell that wafts out of the old fashioned local eateries which sporadically line the streets. I walk by one corner that always had that freshly baked bread smell to discover that it still does. I remember hating walking by this corner in the past as it would instantly make my stomach growl in hunger. I was barely eating when we were living in the truck, and always hungry, there was something about that baked bread smell that would make my stomach lose control every time. I can even feel a twinge from within me right now as I make my way around the corner. I love that smell.

I continue walking keeping my eyes wide and staying alert. I pass the store parking lot where I got jumped that last fateful day that I was here. Everything there still looks the same, except I'm not crawling around on the blacktop spitting up blood. I really hope that I can get this done and make my way back to Evan's car without another episode like that. The old memories make me feel shitty inside, and I have the urge to turn around and run from this place as fast as I can. But I can't.

Finally seeing the old tattered house I make my way to the door and conduct the usual business. No odd looks this time, just straight business as always. I'm happy about the way things went.

Leaving I decide to take a different route back to the truck, just in case someone is waiting for me to walk back through the same way that I came. Also because I want to see another section of the city before I split. I make my way toward the underpass. The rain starts to pick up a little, but it doesn't start pouring. It feels more like a strong mist, and is actually somewhat soothing on the back of my neck. The underpass has a small gathering under it; I assume to stay dry and out of the rain. When you are homeless, you really don't want any of your clothes to get wet – ever. These guys look rough. It's all homeless people here though. No junkies to be seen. No drug activity to be seen for that matter. Just the tattered old boxes and junk that these people use to stay warm in. I walk through the tunnel trying to not feel the depression. I was like this, not this bad, but very close just a few weeks ago. I don't want to be like this. I need to stay focused and stay on the right track for once. My inevitable future is staring right at me underneath this bridge. I don't like it.

I can see the rear taillights of Evan's car, and I'm almost feeling safe. Once inside I lock the doors first thing, and start it up. I made it through the warzone again. I'm starting to feel relief as I get closer to the highway.

The drive to Evan's house seemed long, but was extremely uneventful. I stuck to the speed limits and did my best to obey any special traffic instructions. It still seemed like I had a giant neon sign attached to the roof illuminating the word "HEROIN" when I rolled through a construction site. But I kept my cool, and everything worked out just fine. Evan was happy to see me, and his car, back in one piece when I pulled into the driveway. He jumped in the passenger seat sporting a backpack and we were off to my house – finally.

Evan wanted to know the details of the score. He wanted me to fill him in on the process and how it all goes down. His interest was bursting from his pores as he awaited each answer, which I never really gave him. It's weird to talk about this stuff to someone who isn't in it or doing it. I just know that without being fully involved there's a level of understanding that that person will never get to. You can't. Unless you are living this life that is ruled by the substance itself, none of it really makes any sense. I can describe my addiction using every word in the English language, and it will still be light years from reality. The hold that this shit gets on you is enormous and incomparable to anything else. I give Evan no details whatsoever while trying to appease his curiosity. Besides, if he isn't ever going to use again – then he doesn't need to know. I remind him of this fact as we pull into my driveway.

Nikki is sitting on the couch with three needles lined up in front of her on the coffee table, like we are about to invoke Evan into our secret little club. I tell her to cut the shit and toss her the bag. She gives me a funny look and starts cooking up her hit. It's understood that I'll take care of Evan's. Still feeling very apprehensive about the whole thing I take a seat on floor opposite Nikki. Evan takes a seat to my left and removes his sweatshirt baring his right arm. I start cooking up his dose after seeing Nikki react to hers – it's good stuff, and strong. Taking all of this into account I prepare the needle.

Evan flinches slightly when I push the steel rod into the crook of his arm.

"We're almost there." I whisper, and send him on his way. He has the exact reaction I was expecting. A wide understanding smile spreads across his face, and he nods his head twice. Still looking at me with shock on his face, I get my fix ready. After I ride the initial rush I set the needles down carefully on the table. I lean into Evan and pull him closer by the back of his neck.

"Enjoy it….that was your final hit."

45. Discovered

The next morning is weird. I wake up to Nikki and her mother screaming at each other downstairs. It suddenly feels like I decided to live in a nuthouse. I wonder where her father is and why I don't hear him chiming in from time to time. I wonder what time it is for that matter. I glance over at the alarm clock next to Nikki's bed – its 12:34 – in the afternoon. I climb out of the bed slowly, and limp my way to the bathroom as every muscle in my body is aching out of control. I hear her mother yell something about already getting high. How did she know about the heroin? Nikki must have done something stupid.

I go back to her bedroom to throw on some clothes and she stomps in from the hallway.

"What's going on?" I ask her.

"She came into the room this morning and saw all of our shit on the floor." Nikki barks back at me.

Great. I had no idea that her mother would be busting in on us. The thought had never even crossed my mind. Now I'm going to be pinned as just another junkie in their eyes. Nikki sits down on the bed looking frustrated.

"She said that we can't do it in the house. And to be careful." Nikki mutters in my direction.

"Seriously?"

"Yeah."

"Then why are you so pissed off?" I ask with confusion dripping off of every word.

"Because now I'm going to have to hear about it all the time. She's going to be all nosey and shit."

That was her response. I'm glad that she was still able to find something wrong with this arrangement. I personally saw no need for a fight. Obviously her parents were just going to tolerate whatever behavior she threw at them. Most people would give their right arm for this privilege. Those same people probably wouldn't be exploiting it with drug use either, but that's another story entirely. Her parents were definitely odd, but I thought that we'd be kicked out instantly if they were privy to this information. Apparently I was wrong. We just couldn't use under their roof, which I had my doubts about even being enforced. That sounds like a pretty sweet deal to me.

I wrap Nikki in my arms and tell her to chill out. Everything's all good, no need to fight about anything. Eventually she calms down and everyone is able to coexist once again in peace.

I feel a little weird about seeing her parents now that they have acquired this new knowledge, but both of them seem basically unaffected when I walk down the stairs for the first time. Her father is there sitting in an overstuffed chair in the living room, reading a different book than the one he was so engrossed in last night. Her mother seems to be already hitting the sauce and is actually flipping through the channels on the television. I didn't expect that, but she doesn't seem to really be paying any attention to it either.

They both greet me cheerfully and go right back to doing nothing as if I was just passing through. I suddenly don't feel weird about seeing them anymore. I do feel weird about why, but that's it really. I continue on into the kitchen where I find a bottle of water tucked behind five different bottles of wine in the fridge. I down it quickly, and return to Nikki's bedroom where it's only slightly more normal.

We decide to go out to breakfast at a local diner that doesn't discriminate against people who get up in the afternoon. I love that about diners. You can always count on them to have everything that they serve ready to go as long as their open. On the way over Nikki starts telling me how much she liked the affects of heroin. She goes into this big tirade of how it differs from all of the other drugs she's done. I already know this information, but she feels as though it's important for me to hear it all again. I don't mind listening to her, but I fear that she is going to end up right where I am with it. I fear that she will lust after it with every free moment that she has. I fear that it will replace anything and everything in her life that she cares about and become her number one priority.

I nod at all of her points quietly not really wishing to discuss the topic any further. It still feels weird to me that she used, and that it was my fault. I should have stood my ground and said no. I shouldn't have allowed myself to use again either. I already know the path that I am capable of traveling down. I don't want to do that again. I don't want to overdose and become someone's problem all night long again. I don't want to overdose to the point of death either. I really need to find a way to control this addiction, but I'm already looking forward to the next hit.

We eat our breakfast and fly back to her room as quickly as possible. The physical attraction between us has caused a very urgent distraction which needs to be addressed. Her parents are still in the same configuration when we walk in the front door, but this time her mother has given up on the television and has reverted back to another magazine. Her father smiles at me as we walk up the stairs like he knows everything in detail. He's a very creepy guy. Once in her room the door shuts and Nikki slides a lock over it, which I didn't realize was there. I begin to wonder why she didn't do that last night; but that thought is quickly gone once we fall backwards on her bed. Clothing begins to fly, and starts to become an obstacle so I tear her G-string off with a snap at her hip. This doesn't break her rhythm for a second. Before I know it we are barely even on the bed almost floating in thin air but connected to each other in so many ways. An invisible structure has encased itself around our bodies and we are able to perform impossible stunts with swift precision. The release is powerful and Nikki's head is slammed up against the headboard with such ferocity that the small useless dog downstairs yaps at the sound. We don't really hear this, but we know that it happened. Stuck within our own little world that we've created just for us, everything on the outside seems foreign and very far away. This is another place that I never want to leave. Just like when I'm in the apex of a high. I want to freeze time and keep that feeling forever. It's my ultimate happiness.

We finish and slowly drift back into reality. I realize that I am standing with one foot planted on the ground next to the bed while the rest of my body is still actually on the bed. I feel my uncomfortable stance for the first time and pull myself off of the bed. Flipping through the pile of clothing on the floor I finally find my other lover and pull the wooden box out into view. I set it on the bed and Nikki nods at me with exaggeration. She's ready for round two. So am I. I fix us both up and we get high. Immediately breaking the only rule that has been set forth for us, but I have a very good feeling that the mannequins downstairs won't find out about it this time.

46. Indulgence

It's time for Evan to leave. He has to work later this evening. He's a chef at a local resort that is often frequented by celebrities who decide to vacation in the area. They are fascinated by our ability to grow trees or something, so of all places to travel, they eventually come to this boring spec on the earth. I'll never understand the draw.

Evan hangs around for coffee and gathers his things together so he can hit the road. He never mentions last night to me at. I take this is a good sign. Perhaps he's going to come through on his end of the bargain and walk away with his experience. These are my hopes, and I'm going to hold onto them. I'm going to pretend that last night didn't even exist when it comes to Evan's involvement. I still find myself worrying about it twenty minutes after he leaves. I wish that I could hear his thoughts so that I could know whether or not my concerns had merit. I'll just have to keep tabs on him.

Nikki took a second hit about two hours before Evan and I got up. I saw her do it, but she thought that I was still sleeping. Her dependency hasn't changed since the truck days. She was able to score some shit on her own while I was trying to claw my way out of rehab. She's a tough girl and can take care of herself without any problem at all, but if she has someone to do it for her she'll gladly take a vacation. At her rate the dope is going to be gone in a matter of days. This makes me anxious, but deep down inside the idea of it being gone is comforting. Something has got to give. The water mains are nanoseconds away from bursting. I really can't let things go on like this. I can't run around like a maniac feeding this addiction and destroying others in the process. Nikki needs to face this too. She needs to go to rehab just to dry the fuck out and stay clean for a couple of weeks. Even if she used right afterward her body would at least have those two weeks where she didn't. She's going to kill herself at this rate. It worries me every time I think about her, and I didn't do nearly enough to prevent her from using that very first time. This is on my shoulders. I don't even know where to begin with her now; she's going to go crazy if I even bring up the notion of help.

I am pacing around the apartment and getting all bent out of shape. I feel emotions inside of me traveling up my throat like a geyser. I'm going to cry. It has all gotten to be too much for me to take. I think back to when I was younger and actually experienced happiness in my life. I fast forward to a few years later when I started to wonder why my father had just decided to hit the road once he knew I was on my way. The overwhelming feeling of abandonment swells up in my mouth and my eyes spill over with tears. I sit down on the floor and wrap myself around the legs of the coffee table. Silently crying for another couple of minutes before I am able to shut it all off. I'm drained. I'm tired. I don't give a fuck anymore.

The only thing that will help with the pain right now is sitting on top of the table above me. I can see it through the glass from underneath. In less than a minute I can have it inside of me. I need to fight it. I need to turn and run away in the opposite direction using every single muscle in my body to propel myself at an ungodly speed. I need to pick it up and run into the bathroom with it and flush it down the toilet. I need to lock it away in a welded shut metal box that is impossible to get into. But I can't. And I won't.

I'm on my knees and dumping some out into a metal cap within seconds. Fire, filter, needle, vein. That might have been a record, but I can't be sure. You tend to lose track after the first thousand times doing it. I'm instantly flying and zipping around the room leaving trails of light behind me. The pain was gone before I finished pushing it all in. That alone made it all worth it.

Indulgence

I had to do something to squelch it. I needed to get away. I did a good job. I'm definitely "away".

My head is filled with thoughts of pleasure. Nikki and I wrapped up in each other on the bed. Mountains of heroin that would take 300 years to use up. Gigantic needles with blood pulsing inside of their plastic tubes. Nikki and I fucking on the floor of the kitchen and destroying everything in our path. An entire steak dinner with barrels of mashed potatoes and endless vats of gravy. These are the wonderful thoughts that are swimming around in my head. It's almost as if I'm dreaming while still awake. I am going to take another hit when I start to come down. Just a little taste to throw me back into the grips of the best place on earth. I deserve it. I've been really good since I got out of rehab. I even went and got a job – although I'm not even sure when I have to work again. I suppose that I should check that at some point, but for right now I'm going to enjoy myself and ask questions later.

Nikki walks into the room, which surprises me as I figured she'd be out for another few hours or so. She tells me that it's 5:00pm and gives me an annoyed look. She's cooking up another shot for herself, and it seems as though I've lost almost eight hours. I must have fallen asleep or completely blacked out or something. I have no recollection of even moving let alone being asleep. I tell her to count me in, and we both shoot up simultaneously. I'm not even entirely sure what day it is, nor am I at all concerned. For all I know Nikki and I could have been doing this day in and day out for the last week. It would still seem like it was all the same day to me. Like someone hit pause every time I took a hit.

Nikki is starting to look worse every time I see her. She's getting thinner by the minute and not keeping any food in her system from what I can tell. She has regularly scheduled bathroom visits that occur immediately after eating, and she never has anything in between meals. Her bones look like they could pierce something. This looks especially strange to me when I'm high because my imagination always turns her into a bat for some reason. That's usually when I laugh while staring at her, and she gets annoyed by my unexplainable laughter. I'm not going to tell her that my drugged up brain just turned her into a giant black bat right before my eyes. She would just get more annoyed and think that I was acting retarded, so I just let her get mad and decide not to throw any fuel on the fire.

My wooden box has been permanently propped open on its new home – the coffee table. What used to be a hidden treasure has made its way out into the unprotected living room. Like a stack of books for people to peruse. A sense of accomplishment hits me when I look at it sitting there. It's helping me to keep the negative thoughts out of my head. The little wooden box – out of hiding, and here to stay.

47.   Bottom

Weeks of mayhem ensue. Nikki and I can't keep ourselves out of trouble no matter where we go, and we don't try very hard to avoid it. We embark on a rampage fueled by our incessant heroin use tearing down anything that stood in our way. Money starts to become an issue, but we quickly fix that by stealing everything that we can get our hands on. The contents of the house slowly start to fill up every pawn shop in the area. We eventually run out of things to sell, and decided that jacking the living room furniture would be going too far. Her parents were not happy with our behavior. We finally found a way to piss them off, which I felt somewhat comforting. It didn't seem right for them to simply tolerate everything – that's not what parents are supposed to do.

We spent more and more time hanging out in the magical city just fifteen minutes away by car. I started talking to the other junkies that lived on the streets constantly scouring the area for drugs and money. I started to learn their ways.

One weekend that particularly sucked involved my car getting into an accident right in the middle of town. Some redneck in a giant monster truck ran a red light and basically drove over the front of my car. I didn't even end up with a bruise, but my car was totaled. I was pissed. I had no way to fix it, and no way to replace it. So now the only means of transportation between Nikki and I was her junked up old pick-up truck. It was fine, but it had its own issues. We started really running it into the ground with sudden heavy use because it was all we had. Eventually everything starts to fall apart.

Driving back and forth to the city became a problem the first time that we got pulled over. The truck had a taillight out, which I knew was eventually going to be a problem. The cops around here look for every excuse to execute a traffic stop in hopes of nabbing their catch on something else. They are always looking for that one reason, no matter how benign. We were three miles away from her parent's house when we got stopped. Apparently the cop didn't like how I looked, so he decided that he wanted to search the vehicle, starting with Nikki's purse. That pretty much ended the search. five needles, two of them used and littered with residue, one fresh new packet of heroin, and one fresh smelly bag of weed. We got nailed with possession on two counts. The fucker even wrote us a ticket for the taillight right before he cuffed us both and dragged us off to the station.

Both of us being locked up pretty much left us with nobody to call except for Nikki's parents. They would act all pissed off and disgusted, but ultimately run right down with bail money, so I had no worries about having to stay the night. Nikki gave them a call when we were finally able to use the phone – within two minutes they were on their way down with the cash. They picked us up twenty minutes later, and somehow we were able to get the truck released from the impound lot. We went right back to the city and scored another stash, then made the trip back to her parent's house once again to get high.

Everything was fine once we got back inside the safety of Nikki's room. We did have one problem to think about though. Court the next morning. I started to stress about it. If the judge wanted to I could get thrown in jail on the possession charges, and that means drying out. Drying out the hardcore way with no medical assistance of any kind. This was stressing me out. I cooked up a shot and immediately tried to counteract the worry inside my head. Nikki knew exactly what I was nervous about as well. She was feeling the same way. What were going to do? We can't go to jail. I was terrified to be without heroin. Its absence would be far more damaging to me then my actual physical use. I was convinced of this.

I tried to get my mind off of it by focusing on the moment. Focusing on Nikki and her beautiful long black hair. I looked up at the ceiling fan begging it to cart me off into solitude as it had so many times in the past. Nothing helped. I could hear the drone of the television downstairs that nobody was watching; usually I can find some peace in the background noise, but no luck tonight. My mind was racing around the room thinking about everything all at once. I had no solutions. I felt like a failure.

"We have to get out of here." I tell Nikki while grasping her arm tightly.

"Where? What are you talking about?" She asked bugged eyed.

"Let's load up all of our shit and skip out on court tomorrow. We'll camp out in the city for as long as we can. I'm not going to jail, so if you don't want to come I'll do it myself."

"Let's go"

We ran around the room frantically stuffing things into bags and loading up whatever we thought would be useful. I filled up the wooden box with the essentials and buried it in my backpack taking one final look around the room. Her parents didn't even seem to notice us carrying all the bags down the stairs. Plodding through the snow we made our way to the beat up blue Nissan in the drive way. I jump in the driver seat and take one last look at the house on the gigantic woodsy hill. Nikki gladly climbs in on the passenger side and looks like she's ready to go, so I slowly back out of the driveway and start heading southeast. That, my friends, is how I began waking up every morning in the back of a pick-up truck – homeless, helpless, and completely strung out of my mind.

48. Opinion

Stocking shelves in a non-descriptive aisle toward the rear of the store, I look up and notice my brother walking toward me. I'm moving slowly, but ultimately doing my job with every second that passes, so nobody can really say anything to me about my pace. I wonder how he knew I was working tonight; he must have stopped by the house and figured it out. I wish that I didn't look so high. I took a hit before I walked here a couple of hours ago. Just a small hit to keep me going through the night. My new job has afforded me many luxuries. I couldn't have asked for a better position, unless of course the pay was slightly higher.

I learn that my brother just figured I would be here, so he stopped in looking for me. He wanted to know if I needed anything, and what time I was getting out. I told him midnight and he said that he'd be back to pick me up then. That sounds good to me, looks like I won't have to walk home in the cold tonight. He turns and leaves seemingly disappearing right before my eyes. I return to my stack of boxes and cases of macaroni and cheese dinners. I have about three hours left until I am out of here, and I'm already almost done with this load. I need to go slower. There's nobody here watching me or keeping tabs on me. I just need to have some certain things done before my supervisor comes in tomorrow. I can't run out of things to do, or else I'll lose my mind waiting for the time to pass.

My brother is outside waiting for me when I finally walk out of the store. We make our way out of the parking lot, and then I learn the real reason why my brother picked me up.

"You need to go back to rehab." My brother says to me with a serious look.

"I'm getting things figured out, I'll be fine." I snap back at him. I hate it when I get pestered to go to rehab. He knows that, which means he thought about having this conversation with me for hours before hand. It still irritates me, but the fact that he even wanted to bring it up concerns me. He doesn't look happy with my response, but I don't think he's going to push the issue. When or if the time actually comes that I'll entertain going back to rehab – he'll be the first person that I call, and he knows that too. This sucks though – he must be getting pressured by the entire family. They know that I'm not going to listen to anyone else. I hate being put into these positions.

My brother makes his way to a back road that we loop around on frequently and punches the gas hard. The sudden force throws me back in the seat – my eyes are glued to the radar detector hanging from the windshield. The last thing that he needs is another speeding ticket. That seems to be one of my brother's vices that comes around every once and awhile and bites him in the ass. He lost his license in the first year that he had it for excessive speeding tickets – he hated not being able to drive.

I reach into my pocket and pull out a cassette and pop it into the dash, replacing the one that was playing. My brother gives me another serious look, and then relaxes as soon as he realizes what it is. For some reason we have this bond when it comes to music, and it spans all different genres both old and new. There are a few albums in particular that are always acceptable to be played at any time. This is one of them; we both just lean back in our seats and enjoy the ride. The darkness of the night is soothing, and almost enough to lull me to sleep. I almost wish that I wasn't going back to the apartment.

After what seems like an eternity, my brother decides to bring me home. I reluctantly get out of the car when we get there, and tell him I'll call him tomorrow. Luckily I have the day off. I'm hoping that he'll have time to come over and chill for a little while. It gets a bit depressing being there with Nikki all day long – watching her stuff junk in her veins and flail about the apartment puking every four seconds. I need a change, but I'm not ready. I don't know if I'll ever be ready. My brother was right, but I can't let him know that fully. If I do he'll just pick me up and drive me straight to the nearest rehab. I have to make him believe that I'm not completely fucking up with every move that I make, and that I am actually somewhat trying to get myself out of this rut. I've put everyone through so much shit already; I can't keep hurting the ones who care about me.

Nikki is high as a kite on the couch, pulling a Brad. She's crumpled up in the corner with her face buried in a pillow snoring away. The TV is yelling about some kind of super duty knife set that can cut through your car door if need be. Apparently they are second to the Jaws of Life. Some people must go nuts when they see this shit. It makes me wish that I was more assertive when it came to ripping people off. Then I could just do what these people do, only legally, and make some cash in the process. It's really strange the way the world works. It never ceases to amaze me.

I walk into the kitchen and grab a piece of paper and a pen. I start making a list. I make a list of all the things that I want to change. All of the things that I want to fix. All of the things that I've fucked up and are going to require lots of work and effort. I start writing words down all over the paper in an illegible frenzy. My wrist hurts from the pressure that I apply to the pen. I walk out to the coffee table and drag the wooden box into the kitchen. I want to get away from it but I can't yet. I just simply cannot. I am not able to. I'm like a magnet being pulled with no control of my own to manipulate my course. I need to get high. I need to get more paper. I need to finish this list and actually do something about it. I need to get another pen because this one is bending and is going to break soon. I need to be reborn as somebody else just to avoid ever being sucked in by this terrible substance.

49. Breakdown

Nikki is passed out on the floor face down and barely breathing. Fuck. I've been here so many times before. Having no phone makes things especially interesting. I run outside and across the street to a house that appears to have some life in it. Banging on the door frantically, and shivering to death wearing only a t-shirt and a pair of shorts, I fear that it might be too late. An older lady answers the door reluctantly and I explain to her that I have to call 911 for my friend who might be dying. She lets me in and I find the phone in the kitchen hanging up on the wall without her assistance. I dial 911, tell them the address with urgency, and slam the phone back down. I'm back out across the street before the old lady even realizes that I have already used her phone.

I gently pick Nikki up and cradle her in my arms. She doesn't seem to have overdosed. None of the signs are there. I'm not even sure if she has used recently. The wooden box is still in the kitchen on the counter exactly how I left it early this morning. I put Nikki on the couch and wait for the ambulance to arrive. I pack up all paraphernalia just in case, and hide it all in the closet. Upon closer inspection of the box I can clearly see that I was the last one to have used. This is not an overdose. That's good and bad all at the same time. If it isn't an overdose – what the fuck is it?

I can hear the sirens as the ambulance gets closer. Luckily we are only a few miles from the hospital, so this should be quick. I'll feel a lot better as soon as she is in the paramedic's hands anyways. They load her up on a stretcher and wheel her out to the ambulance, pumping oxygen into her mouth by hand the whole way there. I hop in the back with them and the doors are shut behind us. They ask me if she took anything. I tell them that I don't know, but I don't think so. The two paramedics look at me with disbelief oozing off of their faces. I just shrug my shoulders. I realize that I'm squeezing her hand too hard and loosen my grip. I hate this.

We get to the emergency room and it's time for me to wait while they race her inside and past the triage nurse. She looks up at me, but doesn't seem to recognize me from last year with Brad. Perhaps she does and is just good at hiding it – I can't tell right now. Either way I don't really give a fuck, I just want to know what's wrong with Nikki and why. I sit down in one of the thirty available chairs that are strewn about the waiting room and stare off into space. I'm very impatient when it comes to these situations. Not knowing what is going on drives me completely insane. I just want to go running through the double doors that separate me from all of the dying people and find out what is happening, even if it's nothing. I really hope that they have the consideration to come talk to me as soon as they know something.

Two hours have passed and I am still sitting in the same chair. Staring off into the same space. Still looking at the same nothing. The atmosphere of the waiting room has changed many times in these last two hours. At one point it was almost full, but then it quickly cleared out. The most interesting injury so far was a guy on crutches who seemed to have something sticking out of his leg. It might have even been a piece of bone, but I didn't look at it long enough to find out. He seemed to hobble along without too much trouble, which I found to be quite odd. I know that if something was sticking out of my leg I'd probably be too freaked out to move let along walk with crutches. The other thing that I found to be odd was that he already had crutches. How did that work? Did he hurt himself badly and happen to be in the company of someone who had spare crutches? Was he already on the crutches, which ultimately would help to explain a sudden fall of some sort that caused his bone to break through his skin? I spent about five minutes thinking about his situation. Other than that I have been sitting here doing nothing at all, and dying inside with anxiety. I have spoken to the triage nurse four times, but she has been anything but helpful, almost as if she likes it better that way. Bitch. I fought back the urge to throw a chair through her window. I hate people like that.

Finally after another hour has passed, a doctor comes walking up to me. At first I didn't even bother to lift my head, because I assumed he wasn't there to talk to me. I was wrong however, gladly. He explained to me that Nikki's potassium levels were extremely low and that she may have done permanent damage to some of her organs.

"What has she eaten in the past few days?" The doctor asks me.

"Nothing. She's bulimic and pukes whatever she eats right back up. I've been telling her that she's really going to hurt herself, but she won't listen to me." I reply.

"Ok, well we are going to need to keep her here for a few weeks until she stabilizes, and then we'll seek treatment options afterward to help her deal with the disorder itself." The doctor tells me, trying to sound compassionate.

"Can I see her?" I ask.

"Sure, but only for a few minutes right now, and later tonight she'll get moved to an actual bed in the hospital." The doctor answers while leading me toward the fatal double doors.

She is lying on the stretcher still, and seemingly unconscious. Five bags of fluids are hanging above her head all leading to her arms. She doesn't look good at all. She looks like a limp noodle weighing less than a hundred pounds. I kiss her forehead and make my way back to the waiting room. There's no point in me being here right now, I'll have to come back later after she has her own room. I walk out onto the sidewalk and light up a smoke. Time to make the walk back to the apartment, too bad the truck wasn't back yet. I could have really used it today. I decide to take the long way back home, it's not like I have anywhere special to be, and honestly everything is a little depressing at the moment. I hit up a payphone on the way home and leave my brother a voice mail letting him know what went down today, and that he can swing by whenever if he wants to. Hopefully he doesn't have anything going on later and can find some free time. I'd really enjoy it.

50. Wishful

My brother stopped by a few hours ago. He only stayed for about ten minutes; he already had plans with his girlfriend for the night. It was cool that he stopped in though; he wanted to see how I was doing with everything. I told him that I'd be checking in on Nikki in a little while and that I'd let him know how everything went. He left me twenty bucks in case I needed some cash, and was on his way.

I pace around the apartment trying to figure things out. It has only been a few hours since I left the hospital, so going back there might still be pointless. I'm not really sure what to do. I could give Evan a call and see if he'll come down for a little bit and then bring me over to the hospital later. I'm not sure if I want to pull him into this yet though. It has only been a few days since the monumental night of deflowering Evan's veins. I don't really want him to get any crazy ideas in his head. I decide against contacting him, at least for today.

I prepare myself another dose. It's been almost half a day since I shot up, which seems like some sort of an accomplishment. That's fucked up. I used to think that I'd be able to do this once a week and be all set. I must have been completely insane to have ever believed such a thing. Either insane or just plain stupid, I'm going to go with stupid. Stupid to have not understood the severity of the effects that this drug could have on me. Stupid to ever have thought that I could control it. I was never able to control it. Even in the beginning when I really thought that I was – I wasn't. It has always controlled me. It consumed my every thought from the first time I ever used. I have forever been locked into its grasp. I really have a lot of things to think about before making the final leap to sobriety. These are all the thoughts that I have seconds before taking a hit. Afterward – I couldn't care less.

At least being high will help to pass the time. It will feel like a long time, but the clock will actually continue to move forward, and before I know it an entire block will be filled and gone. Then I can go back to the hospital and find Nikki. I really hope that she is in better condition when I see her. The only upside to this is that she is being forced to stay away from heroin and retain some basic nutrition. I don't have to worry about finding her stuck to the bathroom floor in a pool of her own vomit. I don't have to worry about her passing out and smashing her head into something on the way down. I just have to worry about her getting better while she is in the hospital itself. On some level I need the same exact situation bestowed upon myself. I'm just not ready to do it on my own accord. I'm just not strong enough to face it yet. I hope that I can do something though, before it's too late.

It's 8:00pm and I start to put on some layers to brave the cold. The wind has picked up outside, which has forced me to almost cover my entire face with whatever I can find. This is going to be a brutal walk. On the way there it starts to snow lightly, which inevitably ends up pelting me in the face due to the wind. All I do is concentrate on getting to those automatic doors at the main entrance. Frozen solid, I only have a small parking lot to cross before I'm inside. I make it in and shake all of the frozen bits of snow off of my outer layer.

I can already tell that there are going to be issues at the front desk just by how the lady sitting there looks. She clearly does not want to be bothered, and has taken this job only because of the time in which it occurs. During the later hours around here nothing much really happens at the main entrance to the hospital. I would bet that she ends up talking to about two people per night. Ironically this job sounds like heaven to me, it's exactly what I'd want to do, but she looks pissed to even have to deal with one person. She's worse that I am. I didn't think that was possible. I stand my ground and walk right up to her like she owes me something and ask where Nikki is. Fighting the urge to be a bitch, she responds through gritted teeth "Room 310." I continue walking down the hallway to the elevators.

That wasn't as bad as I had originally anticipated. Once on the third floor I walk through the maze of tiny numbered signs twice before I understand their configuration. Room 310 is all the way down a hall across from a vending area. I try to find some convenience in that, but come up with nothing.

She is in bed one and has a neighbor in the room with her occupying the window portion of the room. It's all I can do to keep my eyes from staring at the bloodied bandaged leg of the patient in bed two. It's just too realistic for me; I have to pretend that it isn't there. Nikki herself looks exactly the same as when I saw her earlier – just hooked up to more machines now. I count six bags, this time, hanging from various metal trees scattered around her bed. The electronic monitors seem to be working normally and not reporting any clear danger. She is still unconscious. The nurse on duty flitted in and out of the room a few times just to check in on everything. She informs me that normal visiting hours are over, but I can stay there as long as I want. So I sit in the chair by her bed. I don't bother lifting up the attached television remote that is dangling from her bed. I just sit there in the darkness listening to the quiet beeps of the machines. The neighbor in bed two also shows no interest in the TV, so the quietness is still and soothing.

I started to think back to the way things used to be. The way that things used to be with her and I, and how I had thought that finally I had found my place. I had found the person that I wanted to be with forever, no matter what happened. I had found the person whose face lit up with joy every time she saw me. I fear that our common interests and similar personalities have ultimately destroyed our relationship. They have destroyed whatever relationship we would have been able to create, not even having a fair chance in the first place. The really upsetting thing about this is that we both allowed it to happen. We both gave in to our addictions above everything else, and drove our own way into this mouth of destruction. All of it was preventable. That's what bothers me the most.

I sat there holding her hand, hoping that at any moment she would wake up and be the person that I knew she was on the inside. I hoped that this time she'd realize she had gone too far, and would work to get everything that was lost back. This time she'll come to grips with reality and be scared to let anything else happen to herself or us. I just want her to get through this, and ultimately be clean afterward, otherwise there isn't going to be an afterward – for either of us. The thought of her being hurt breaks my heart and tears me apart inside. I can't stop blaming myself for dragging her down my self-destructive path. I only hope that one day she'll forgive me for all of the damage that I have done.

51. As Usual

My shoulders feel like they have been crumpled up into balls of foil from a giant pair of hands. I wake up in the wooden chair next to Nikki's bed. The sun is shining in from the large window across the room. I have no idea what time it is. 10:30am on the nose according to the institutional looking clock that is hanging on the wall in between the two beds. I once again try to concentrate on not looking at the neighbor's ripped up leg. It's guaranteed to look even more horrid now that there is natural light in here. I'll lose it if I get a good look at it.

Nikki reaches over to my arm and grasps it lightly with her fragile boney fingers. They feel like little needles trying to twist their way around my skin. There is nothing left to her at all. She has literally whittled herself down to that of a skeleton. I look into her sunken eyes, and she gives me an understanding look. We haven't even had a conversation yet about why she is here, or what happened, and to the best of my knowledge this is the first time that she has been conscious since I brought her here. But she knows somehow. She knows why she is here, and is actually showing a small thread of remorse as she stares back at me from the bed. I want to reach out and hold on to this feeling for as long as I can, so that I can pull it out and show it to her later on when she decides to be completely unreasonable. I want to lock us into this mood forever, and leave everything else behind. I'm ready to do it with her – if only she'll join me. I continue to stare at her in silence, overjoyed inside that she is actually awake once again.

The nurse comes in a few minutes later and is also very happy that Nikki is awake. She explains to her that she needs to be monitored for a few more days because of the dangerously low nutrient levels that they found in her blood. Damage to her kidneys, heart, and liver has become an immediate concern, and they need to be really careful with her diet while she is there. Nikki smiles and nods at the nurse convincingly, and then gives me a dirty look when she isn't looking. Obviously she isn't going to fully cooperate with the treatment plan. I cross my arms and look sternly back at her trying to be intimidating, this just makes her more frustrated. The nurse leaves finally, and Nikki starts climbing out of bed.

"Where are you going?" I ask her.

"To the bathroom, and I have to do something about my hair while I'm in there so give me a minute." She replies while grabbing her purse on the way to the door.

I sit there waiting, not thinking anything suspicious really; I'm the one that brought her here so I know everything that she has in that purse. I keep my eyes away from the neighbor while I wait and stare at random objects throughout the room. Suddenly I smell the very faint odor of smoke. Cigarette smoke. That's what she wanted to do in the bathroom! I jump up and try opening the door, but it's locked, and she won't let me in.

"Hey. You can't do that in here what are you nuts?" I whisper as loudly as I can up against the door. I can only make out muffled noises coming from the other side mixed with sounds of water being turned on and off randomly. After about five minutes she comes out and a wave of smoke and air freshener hits me in the face. Since these facilities are so extremely smoke free, that's all you can smell when someone breaks the rules. As soon as the next nurse comes in here Nikki is busted. They might even move her to another floor to keep better tabs on her. I have no clue why she would actually entertain doing what she just did in there. Sometimes she makes the most stupid decisions.

She smiles at me as she walks by and climbs back into bed rolling her little metal trees along with her every step. I sit back down in the chair and shake my head slowly, not even knowing what to say to her. It's not like anything is going to make a difference, she just does whatever she wants no matter what anyway.

The nurse comes in and at first doesn't say anything, whether she notices the smell and is being cool about it, or she actually doesn't notice it is unclear. Then she notices Nikki's heart monitor, which has increased in speed quite a bit. The nurse decides to further investigate and pulls out her stethoscope to listen to Nikki's heart. With a puzzled look on her face she moves around her chest listening for an issue, but seemingly finding nothing. Then a light bulb goes on, I watch as her face lights up ever so slightly, and then a look of frustration sets in. She looks around the room carefully, trying to find the evidence and walks over to Nikki's purse as if it had an arrow hanging above it. Right on top of the open purse, just barely tucked inside the two flaps, is a pack of smokes. She pulls them out and looks at Nikki.

"Did you just smoke?"

"No" Nikki replies with disgust plastered all over her face. The nurse walks into the bathroom and then right back out again after about two seconds.

"Yes you did. And you did it in there." The nurse says pointing toward the bathroom. "These are staying with me for now" while shaking the pack, then looking at me "And please don't bring her anymore." She turns and walks out of the room.

Already Nikki has started to make a reputation for herself here. She's been awake for about twenty minutes and the nurse on duty already has her pinned for trouble, and she'll make sure that everyone else on the floor knows that as well. It should make things very uncomfortable when Nikki starts drying out from withdrawal and can't seem to get any junkie compassion from the staff. This detox might be just as bad as my stint in jail a few weeks ago, because these people are not going to take any pity on her in the least. I hope for her sake that I'm wrong, but I fear that I'm not. I get up and tell her that I'm going to run back to the house to shower.

"I have to work later, but I'll come spend the night again when I get out." I tell her as I lean in and kiss her on the forehead. She strains her muscles to force out a smile, and I turn toward the door once again avoiding the patient in bed two. I'm going to get a good look at that leg one of these days I just know it, and I'm really afraid as to what my reaction is going to be. I hate hospitals.

Finding my way back out the front doors is almost impossible. The elevator buttons confuse me and I end up going to three different floors before hitting the right one. At some point they decided to set everything up with letters rather than numbers, and that really fucks me up when I am trying to navigate multiple floors of a building. M, G, C, L. I don't get it. M could be Main. L could be Lobby. G could be ground. I assume that C is cafeteria, but who knows I probably have that one completely wrong as well. It's probably actually Cathedral or something else light years away from what I actually think it should be. I wish that I could just hop in from the third floor and hit 1. But that doesn't work. G is too far down, L makes no sense to me at all when the doors open, and I finally get it with M, which must ultimately stand for Main. With sufficient confusion occupying all of the remaining space in my head, I walk a straight line to the automatic doors, and feel lucky to have gotten out alive.

52.   Round Two

Evan is waiting at my house when I show up. He's camped out in the driveway. I contemplate for a minute taking off down the road before he could see me and avoiding the situation altogether, but I ultimately walk up to the driver's side door. He rolls down the window and shoots me a look that I've seen before. He wants to use. He's not tearing his skin off with craving, but he definitely wants to use again. I have no clue as to how to deal with this right now. I motion him to come inside. He gets out of the car and follows me in the house without saying a word.

Once inside I explain the Nikki situation to him. He shows his concern and then goes into this long explanation about how the resort he works for is sending him off to California for two weeks to attend some sort of cooking seminar. He figured that since I already had stuff and that he wasn't even going to be around for the next couple of weeks he'd try to get high one last time before blowing town. I wasn't expecting this type of attack, and was caught completely off guard. I stuck to my guns at first and then folded quickly the minute he challenged me. It's so hard for me to stand in someone's way. I put myself in their shoes and immediately have trouble continuing to say no. It's just another one of my weaknesses.

I reiterate the special circumstances to him while I drag the little wooden box out to the living room. He seems completely calm and collected, and nods when I tell him that the only reason why I'm giving in is because I don't believe that he has any kind of a problem yet. This is true. I actually think that he's still outside of the giant lasso that this drug spawns. I am however more and more worried about the future. Every small step in that direction increases the chances of its hold exponentially. It's only a matter of time until it winds itself around every skin cell on your body, and it doesn't take long.

Done with my speech, I hook us both up and send Evan on a still new, but now slightly more familiar ride. The second time using is just as special as the first, but in very different ways. The first time takes you by storm and surprises you with every minute that passes. It's almost too much. The second time however, you have a better idea as to what to expect. This allows the user to really experience the high and relax a little bit. I felt like an expert the second time that I used, that's how much different the experience itself was. By the third time you are actually very anxious because you feel extremely prepared. Eventually you find yourself doing it simply to stay alive, that's pretty much where I am again, stabilizing myself with each subsequent hit that I take. Higher dosage. Higher frequency.

Evan slides into the corner of the couch as I slowly pace around the room again trying to think clearly. I have the entire afternoon still before I need to start getting ready for work. Tonight is going to be long. I have no desire at all to go in to work, but I know that I have to. I know that I can't just keep fucking off whenever I want, or I'll end up losing this job too. I really don't want that to happen. Seeing as how I actually don't mind this job, I'd love to not lose it within a week of starting. For now I'll do whatever I can to keep it for as long as possible.

Nikki is obviously going to be in the hospital for awhile. I 'm going to have to figure something out about dope soon too, I'm getting dangerously low. First I have to find some more cash. I'll be getting a little bit of money from working last week, but it was only for a couple of days and really won't be for much at all. I need more in order to make the trip to the city beneficial. Just at that moment a light bulb inside of me turns on with an explosion. If Evan is going to California for two weeks that means he won't need his car. I wonder if he'll let me use it while he's gone. Hopefully he wakes up within the next six hours or so.

Hopefully I won't have to bribe him too much to get the car either.

I scour the kitchen for food in hopes that there will be something easy and quick to shove down my throat. It feels like I haven't eaten in days and truth I may not have actually. I remember having a small bag of chips the other night while I was at work; I found them in the stockroom and decided that their new home was my stomach. I try to save cash whenever I can. I am slowly building an empire here after all. My stomach is empty, and my hands are starting to quiver from malnutrition. I grab onto the counter and stabilize myself for a minute. The fridge is just as bare as the rest of the kitchen, but I am able to find some cheese that surprisingly has not spoiled yet. I slide down onto the kitchen floor with my new found prize and enjoy its creamy goodness. I had forgotten what it tasted like, which makes me laugh a little.

Hours pass as I find myself in the same position, leaning up against the fridge. I look down at my hands and the cheese is gone – I must have eaten it. Evan is still slumped over on the couch as I walk through the living room in a daze. I should really start getting ready for work; it must be getting close because the sun is almost down. I slowly make my way to the shower, stopping by the heap of clothes in the bedroom on my way. The water feels good and aids in bringing me to my senses. I could stand here all day long providing that the water would just stay hot. It makes me want to never go outside again, at least not while its twenty degrees out.

I am forced to roust Evan to his feet. He seems very surprised at the time, but agrees to drop me off at work before he goes back home. On the ride over I bring up my plan of borrowing his car while he's gone. He agrees to my plan without even blinking an eye. I didn't really anticipate much of a struggle, but I didn't expect him to be that agreeable. He's leaving in two days, and it all works out better this way anyways, because I'll be the one that drives him to the airport. Then I'll have transportation for two weeks straight. That's going to feel great.

I walk into work only fifteen minutes late, and luckily I don't think that anyone has even noticed. This store has a slightly slower paced atmosphere than the one across town that I used to work at. Things don't seem to be so carved out of stone when it comes to rules and regulations. The other store was like working in an area that was under constant surveillance, with a behavioral specialist manning all of the monitors. They would sit and wait for you to do anything against protocol, and then swoop down on you like a hawk. I hated that feeling, and I certainly hated all of the bullshit that went along with that kind of environment. It's not like that here. Sure you are going to get talked to if you fuck off all the time and clearly show no regard for your job, but that's where it ends. If you come in and actually give somewhat of a shit – the small things are let go. I wish that more people had the luxury to know what that feels like.

53. Failing

I spend another night in the chair by Nikki's bed, but she doesn't even seem to really care. I decide that I'm going to stay away from her for a few days. This schedule is starting to get a bit daunting anyways, so it's for the best. She doesn't want to be in the hospital anymore, but she has no choice. She's detoxing like crazy and is very pissed off about it. The meds that they are giving her aren't helping as much as they usually do, so the process isn't going very well. She's irate all the time, and completely intolerant of just about anything. I feel as though a break will be good for us. Give her some time to deal with the immediate withdrawal. I still have no idea what is in store for her once she gets out of here. I would imagine that they are going to try to push her in the direction of rehab. I really don't want to be around for that conversation.

Navigating my way out of the hospital again I'm back out on the street on foot, and headed toward the apartment. Work was slow last night, but didn't present any obstacles, which was nice. The night flowed as it should have, and I was barely bothered at all, not even by customers. It was as if I wasn't even there most of the time. I find this quality to be monumental in why I continue to show up each time I am scheduled. So far I haven't missed a single day. One week down – we'll see what happens next week.

I'm back at the apartment once again. Finally alone and to myself without the unnecessary stimulation of others, sometimes it feels good to be alone with my thoughts. Every day is starting to seem like a repeat to me. Things are just like when I was living out of the truck, only less dangerous. I feel like I am not really getting anywhere with anything. The work part is good, but it's not enough. I have settled. I have basically given up on bettering myself, and have settled to perform even less than required. The job is just a disguise to make me believe that I am "doing the right things". Who am I actually kidding though? Apparently myself, and even that's not working anymore, because I don't buy it.

One more day though and I have Evan's car. I'm planning on running to the magical city and scoring some more shit, but not until I grab some cash from someone. I need to call in a favor – if I have any left. Off of the top of my head I can't seem to come up with anything, so I'm going to have to dig really deep and see what comes my way. I search all of the usual hiding spots in the house to ensure that there isn't anything stashed away that I don't know about. I end up finding a 20 dollar bill stuffed inside an odd container on the floor of the closet in the bedroom. At least the search turned up something and didn't leave me completely empty handed. Now that I have accomplished at least one thing that points me in the right direction – it's time for a dose.

I waited it out this time for a few hours before allowing myself to get a fix. I am trying to wean myself back as much as possible, hopefully that will help to aid in an actual transition to sobriety in the near future. Ever since my brother told me to go back to rehab it has been on my mind night and day. I struggle with the idea of going back there again, and whether or not it will even help. I am having trouble pushing myself toward actually making that leap. I can't do it yet. I am not physically capable. I can't picture myself surrounded by those muted colors and zombie like people. I can't think about that awful coffee pot that sits on the banquet table in the common area all day long. I can't imprison myself there – not even in my mind – without feeling a wave of insanity. The staff with their theories. The meds and tiny cups of water. The little games that are strewn about the tables and couches. I can't make myself willingly walk back into that setting. A team of monster trucks equipped with the heaviest chains are going to be needed to drag me down the street while I claw my way in the other direction. It scares me more than dying at this point.

I think about going to rehab every time before I use. I think about it while I am preparing the dose, and spiking my vein. But I can't stop. I can't put it all down and walk away on my own accord. I never used to think about stopping, so perhaps that's a good sign, but the process itself is driving me out of my mind. When I wake up from each drug induced coma, within five minutes, I am overridden with guilt for not being able to stop. I am burdened with a forever feeling of failure, and no clear end in sight toward success. Sometimes I believe that not existing at all is a much better alternative. If only I had enough gall to pull that stunt. I've thought about it before, but never for long – it's not something that I would be able to go through with. No matter how peaceful or appealing the outcome sounds to me.

I push the fluid into my veins, and lean my head back in relief. The feeling has returned, and is finally taking over for awhile. My breathing becomes extremely labored, and I immediately know what has happened. I did it again. I took too much. Fuck. There's nothing that I can do except to wait and see what happens. Fatal or not, I'm about to be useless in ten seconds anyways, so it's somewhat irrelevant. I drop to the floor and concentrate on air flow. My lungs have been deflated to long rubber flaps fluttering around in my chest and striving for oxygen. My strength is gone, and feels as though it will never return. My eyes are stapled shut and unable to open. My limbs are glued to the floor. I'm still alive, or I'm already dead – there's no way for me to be certain at this time. I have to wait.

54. Assistance

The couch feels like a bed of nails against my body. The pain is unbearable, and I wish that I could take another hit just to make it go away. My brother is sitting next to me staring off into space while quietly smoking a cigarette. I remember bits and pieces that transpired from yesterday morning until now, but for the most part it's as if somebody hit fast forward on the entire episode. I suppose that's a good thing, suffering through it in real time must be horrible. My brother realizes that I am awake and asks me how I am feeling. I tell him that I hurt like hell, but otherwise I just feel tired.

As it was explained to me, my brother managed to break the lock on the door knob of the front door in order to get to me. The deadbolt was left unharmed so closing the door won't be a problem. He pulled me to my feet when he got here and propped me up on the couch to monitor my breathing as best he could. He stayed with me through the night and just hung out in the living room apparently watching infomercials throughout the night. I had puked all over the place at some point, but my brother cleaned everything up. I was surprised about that because he's not very good with vomit situations. I remember back to when we were young and whenever someone would get sick he'd disappear. He couldn't even handle hanging around long enough to hear the sounds. The fact that he dealt with my mess will not be forgotten.

I feel like the most useless retard in the world sitting here on the couch coming out of an overdose while my brother waits by my side having a smoke. These are things that we already barely discuss, and now he has to see me in this fragile strung out state. I hate it. I want to go outside and crawl through the blacktop until I have dug a tunnel all the way to the center of the earth. I want to snap my fingers and be on the other side of the world thousands of miles away. But instead I sit here and continue to face my fears.

"Seriously man." My brother stares from the other side of the couch.

" I know, I know, I'm working on it." I shoot back at him.

We both turn back toward the television screen, neither of us interested in the content. I am trying to break the tension, so I go out to the kitchen and find an old bottle of brandy that I think was left here by the previous tenants. Scraping up two clean cups for the brandy was quite a chore. More of a chore than I expected. I end up finding a coffee mug and a bright red party cup that appeared to be clean. I'll use the red cup just in case it's dirty. I pour us both a shot and sit back down on the couch. My brother goes right for it and lights another smoke. I grab one from my pack and make my own contribution to the polluted air. We sit there in silence for a long time. It wasn't exactly uncomfortable, just slightly odd.

Tonight I'm supposed to bring Evan to the airport so that I can drive back here with his car, but I am clearly in no condition to pull of such a task. I'm drained from yesterday's episode and can barely move fifteen feet without holding onto something. The pain in my muscles and joints is excruciating with every step, and I can't stay drunk enough to drown it out completely. My brother offers to bring Evan to the airport for me, that way I can stay here and chill and still get his car for the two weeks that he's gone. He is also going to stop into the hospital really quick to check on Nikki, just to let her know that everything is ok, and that I'll be up in a couple of days or so. Evan should be here in about twenty minutes.

"I'm going to stop and grab smokes on the way back. You getting low?" My brother asks me.

"Yeah I could definitely use a pack – get the menthols this time though, I have a craving." I respond, glad that the silence has been broken finally. I don't like it when things are weird between the two of us. It just seems strange. It's only when it comes to heroin though. That's the only thing that affects our communication. I don't talk about it, because I don't like to. It's not something that I am proud of, and I never will be. Maybe one day when I have successfully kissed it all goodbye I'll be able to more fully open up about my addiction with the people who care about me. Right now it's far too painful for me to handle. I say what needs to be said and nothing more. I keep it simple, and try to keep my loved ones as far away from the reality of it as possible. It isn't their life and therefore isn't their problem. I usually welcome any help that comes my way, but for the most part I don't expect it. Deep down inside I know that I don't deserve it in the first place. The people who decide to be responsible in this world are always the ones who get punished in the long run. I hate knowing that I contribute to that. Taking one look at my brother is a good reminder. He does all the things that are seen as necessary in society – enough to take care of himself and the people around him. No matter what he'll always be able to find his way without much aid from others. I on the other hand have the same skill, but I lack the assertiveness. I take care of myself in all the wrong ways. I make sure that I have a fresh supply of dope before I dare waste an entire night at work. I start scheming every morning thinking of ways to get more money at the expense of others to help pad my own insufficient income. My motives are different, and for some reason always surround what I shouldn't be doing. Always choosing the road that is wrong, bad, or illegal. All for the escape from reality, which ultimately is the source of all my pain.

Evan shows up and understands that I'm not in very good shape. He doesn't know that I overdosed, but I assume that my brother will discreetly fill him in on the ride out to the airport. I hope that he does just to put a scare into Evan. Evan's heroin use is not known by anybody at the moment except for Nikki and me. If my brother knew I think he'd be really unhappy. It's bad enough that he has to deal with the constant reminder of Nikki's presence in my life which directly contributes to my heroin addiction. He knows that Nikki is a force in my life that holds me back on some level. I'm powerless over her, and I've accepted that fact.

We all chill in the living room for about fifteen minutes and then the two of them get up to leave.

"I'll be back in about three hours. Here's my cell, hit my pager if there's any kind of emergency. Otherwise I'll see you then." My brother tosses me his phone.

"Sounds good, thanks again for doing this." I nod toward them, and the door closes behind them.

55. Coping

My brother returns right on time with Evan's car, and decides to come inside for a little while before leaving. I'm still feeling pretty shitty about myself for allowing things to get where they are right now. I feel like I can't do anything on my own anymore. I always need help from others, which is fine, but its due to my addiction – it always is. I fuck things up and can't manage on my own. Something has to be done.

I ask my brother if he can give me a ride down the street to the package store so that he can buy me a couple 40's. It's the cheapest, largest amount of alcohol I can get my hands on. If I have to stoop low enough to ask my brother for money, I will at least make the amount as small and necessary as possible. He agrees, and we take a trip in Evan's car. My brother throws me a ten dollar bill when we pull up to the liquor store and tells me to get as much as I can. I wasn't expecting that – but I'll take it.

This particular liquor store doesn't get much local business. It sits on a frequently traveled route that is a straight shot into the neighboring state. The state lines meet in a very rural area. Woods everywhere and not a lot of development as you traverse from small town to small town. This particular liquor store is pretty much in the middle of nowhere. This affords me some opportunity. The inside is a bit dungy and clearly hasn't changed in fifty years. It has not been updated and converted into the more conventional wide open layout that you would expect of a normal liquor store. There are plenty of small nooks and crannies to get lost in with racks randomly placed throughout the main part of the store. The lighting is very dim inside, which usually makes it look closed from the outside. There is always either the same old man, or old woman running the register, and other than that, nobody else to be found. I have actually never seen anyone else working there. After going there for years you get to really know what you can or can't get away with depending on the day. I hope that today ends up being like the last five times that I was here.

I walk in the front door and immediately hear the old cow bell that's attached to the swinging arm which allows the door to open. The old guy behind the register to my right acknowledges me with a nod and immediately drops his head back to a newspaper. I smile innocently at him and head toward the cooler doors that line the rear of the store. Luckily for me, the specific section of cooler that holds my interest is conveniently blocked from view by a large rack of wine that stands right in front of it. Lifting shit from here is almost too easy, and sometimes even makes me feel bad. I can't seem to help myself though, it's just too easy. I open up the door and start setting cold 40's on the ground in front of me. After setting two down I pull two more out of the cooler, one in each hand, and watch them respectively disappear down both of my pant legs – one in each side. My pants are equipped for this type of operation, and I have discreetly tucked the excess denim into my shoes so that the bottles can't fall out the bottom. I pull two more out of the cooler and cradle them in my arms while scooping the other two on the floor up carefully. I make my way up to the counter and set the 40's down in front of the old guy. He reluctantly picks his head up from the newspaper to ring up my purchase and packs it all up in a large paper bag, never once showing even an ounce of suspicion toward me. The total comes to $9.60, and I walk out with six 40's in total. Not really a big deal, but every little bit helps.

My brother rolls his eyes at me as I unload my "purchases" from my pant legs once I get back in the car. He isn't surprised, but perhaps he just didn't think that I would do something like that today. Either way it doesn't really make a difference. We drive back to the apartment and hang out in the living room for another hour or so before my brother hits the road for the night.

I really want to go visit Nikki, but I don't want to visit the girl that's lying there in room 310. I want to visit the real Nikki that is locked away inside of her not able to claw her way through the drug that is controlling her mind. I want just one last chance for the two of us to be together without all of the bullshit. I want us to have that, I think that on some level I deserve it, but then the more I think about it, I feel as though I don't deserve it at all. I have made all of my decisions on my own, and need to take responsibility for that. Others might not have helped all that much, but it's still my fault ultimately and not theirs. I decide to take one more night away from her before going back to the hospital. It's not easy to stay away at all, but I think it's for the best right now.

I've already gone through three of the 40's by the time I realize that they are half gone. The clock is nearing 2:00am. I need to slow down on the alcohol or I'm going to be out before I know it. All I have stashed up for the run to the city is 80 bucks which isn't going to get me a whole lot of shit, so I don't really want to piss any of it away on beer, but I might have to. I start scheming again while sitting there staring at the infomercials. I am desperately trying to think of ways to scare up some money. Just another 50 bucks or so would be perfect. Maybe I can convince the store to give me an advance. I then quickly give this some thought, and realize that I'm being completely unrealistic. I've been there for a week, they don't know me at all yet, I'm usually late, and it's a complete shit job. They probably aren't going to give me a cash advance on my pay. I give up at about 2:30am and finish off a fourth giant beer. I was never a drinker at all really, but lately I have been turning to alcohol more and more in order to cope with the undesirable affects from heroin use. It also helps me with some of the withdrawal symptoms. I can go longer in between hits if I keep myself loaded up with alcohol. It takes the edge off just enough that the cravings are easier to deal with. At least I am trying something to curve my habit, even I'm still completely unable to control it or give it up. I allow myself to pass out on the couch after making certain that the cigarette I just smoked is completely out in the ashtray on the coffee table.

56. Desperation

I have shut out as much of the outside world as possible these last few weeks. My job is gone – I only know this information because of my brother. He's the only person that I bother to answer the door for anymore – and even that takes a lot. The store has his cell phone number down as a point of contact. After not hearing from me for three days they left him a voice mail saying that I was terminated. I sit in this empty house all day long, sometimes for eight hour clips without even walking into another room. I have no desire to move, and no desire to speak. I have failed with cutting back my dope use – as usual. Nikki called in a favor with her parents from her hospital bed and managed to score a chunk of cash. She buried the envelope in a flower pot that she asked my brother to bring to the apartment. A sealed hand written letter from her was stuck in the soil – her map to the money was inside. I made a trip to the city with every dime that I was able to scrape up along with the flower pot stash and turned it all into dope. That was last week some time. Evan came and got his car with the help of my brother the other day. All I said to him was "hi" and then I went back to staring at the coffee table. He left quickly and without saying a word to me. Perhaps that is why everyone in my life has disappeared – I push them away. It doesn't matter anymore – heroin is killing me – and I know it. That's not even the worst part. The worst part is that I can't stop. When I die my rotten corpse of a hand is going to claw its way to the surface just to score more dope. I'm close to giving up.

My brother keeps trying to talk to me – I can tell. He doesn't stay very long when he's here, because he knows that I just want to be alone. There are moments when I know that he wants to say something, but he doesn't. I know that he wants to drag me out of the apartment by my hair and hurl me toward safety, but he doesn't, because he knows that I won't comply. He's dealing with a lot right now when it comes to me, but I am physically incapable of helping him. I have failed in so many ways.

Nikki is still in the hospital. She has had a few episodes during her stay there. Her body has been through the war between the bulimia and the heroin use. During the detox period she was in danger of cardiac arrest from the damage that her heart has sustained. Certain meds that she was on have conflicted with others and her body just wants to give up. According to my brother she has been in the clear for the past two days, but they don't feel comfortable letting her out yet. She'll be going straight to rehab when she does get out though – apparently some of the doctors and nurses have been able to slowly talk her into it over the last few weeks. She has gotten much more reasonable with the drugs finally out of her system. I'd love to go see her, but I just can't find the strength to leave the apartment.

If it wasn't for my brother I would have died of starvation at this point. Lack of food would never have been enough to get me out of this house. Only one thing has been successful in that respect so far and that trip was terrible. I didn't think that I was even going to make it back without hitting something on the highway. I ended up going about sixty in the slow lane the entire way home. For the most part traffic avoided me. It wasn't pretty.

Things that my brother knows I'll eat started showing up every time he'd visit. I have barely eaten anything, but apparently just enough to stay alive. Out of desperation and sheer necessity I would take a bite of something that he left for me before returning to whatever corner of the room I was occupying at that time. The fridge has almost become stocked with food that he's brought over in the last week or so, but I can't bring myself to eat any of it. My stomach hurts all the time and never feels quite right no matter what I do to it. My body is really starting to feel the wear and tear from using. It feels as though it is rebelling against itself with every movement. So far I have been unable to find anything that helps with the pain other than more heroin.

Drinking like a fish helps a little bit, but only to a certain extent. I always end up back at the needle. My joints have been replaced with chalk, or so it seems. Every step sends a ripple of pain through my body. As the day progresses I'll get slightly more mobile, but the aching never fully goes away. Morning brings it all back again full force. Standing for the first time is quite the chore and takes a little bit of work. My head pounds at random times, which leaves me with a permanent headache. My lips seem to be the only thing on my body that doesn't hurt all the time.

My family is keeping their distance at the moment. I haven't talked to my mother in over a week. Some messages have been relayed with help of my brother, but other than that I've really secluded myself. I have no idea how to pull myself out of this slump. I don't remember the last time I felt this desperate and hopeless. It wasn't even this bad when I was homeless and conducting my life from the back of a truck. I'm going to need help getting out of this. There's no way that I'm going to be able to do it on my own. I can't even think far enough into the future to know what steps to take. I don't care enough, and have no idea when I ever will again.

57. Change

The banging on the door just won't seem to go away. I keep telling myself that if I just close my eyes and wait a little longer it will disappear – but it never does. I give in, and hobble over to the front door. My brother walks in complaining about having to wait so long for me to come to my senses. He walks past me and straight into the bedroom. I follow behind him, but at about a quarter of the speed. As I get closer I can see that he is throwing clothes into bags and tossing them on the bed.

"What are you doing?" I ask trying to sound as irritated as I can.

"You are getting out of here this morning, whether you like it or not. I'm bringing you to Jeremy's house." He replied in a triumphant tone.

Jeremy is a friend of mine that has been around for years. I don't even remember how I met him, but I'm sure that it was due to strange events. Jeremy was a few years older than me, but he always acted like he was stuck in his early twenties. He never really got into trouble or anything like that, but his mentality just seemed a bit more immature than the rest of us. He works for a flooring company, and he has had this same job for about fifteen years or so. Every day he is either stapling down carpet in an office, or tiling a rich person's bathroom. He's always happy and loves to just hang out and drink during his off time. Jeremy can get annoying at times, but he's a lot easier to deal with than most people.

"Wait, wait, wait, I'm not drying out or anything like that. If that's your plan you can leave now." I say to my brother.

"Did I say that? You need to get out of this place, and you need to actually be around another living person. We can deal with the rest of it when the time comes." He replied.

In a lot of ways I am dreading this. I don't see the purpose for arguing though. I won't win, no matter what I do, so I don't really see the point. He already has the majority of my things packed and ready to go. I go to the closet and grab my backpack which always gets filled with the essentials. The first thing to pack is the little wooden box that is sitting on the coffee table. Looks like it's time for it to find a new home. I love that thing.

My brother has all of the rest of the bags loaded in his car by the time I put the last thing into my backpack. It appears as though we are ready to go. I take one last scan around the room to make sure that I 'm not forgetting anything important and follow him out to the car.

It's only a fifteen minute drive to Jeremy's place from here. Ironically he lives about half a mile away from the liquor store that I often frequent, it's funny how some things in life work out. I'm sure I'll find this new location extremely convenient. The only problem is that I'm farther from everything else now. I can't just walk into downtown. I can't walk to the hospital from here – it would take too long. So now I am going to have to rely on rides from other people, or find a way to get my hands on Nikki's truck if it ever finds its way out of the shop. There have been a whole bunch of runarounds at the shop apparently, so its repairs have been delayed. There has also been talk of Nikki's father keeping the truck when it was fixed. That would suck.

Jeremy isn't home, but apparently that doesn't matter as my brother already has a key to the house on his key chain. He unlocks the door and I walk into the small quiet house. Jeremy actually has furniture strewn about like a normal house, clearly someone actually lives here. There's a large wire cage in the corner of the kitchen that seems to be housing a chinchilla. That's pretty cool yet odd at the same time. There are a couple empty pizza boxes stacked on top of each other on the kitchen table. A few stacks of mail here and there can be seen. Other than just that little bit of random clutter, the house is quite clean and comfortably lived in. Jeremy lives here alone and there are two spare rooms in the back, so he has plenty of room. I peek into his bedroom and a lazy golden retriever is sleeping on his bed. She lifts her head slowly and starts wagging her tail without getting up. It's strangely homey here. I might actually not mind it as much as I had originally thought.

"Jeremy knows that you are going to be here when he gets home today from work. Feel free to do whatever, oh and check this out." My brother motions me to follow him out to the back porch.

The back porch is completely closed in with a couple of windows on one side that face a decent sized backyard which fades into woods. There are no neighbors for 200 feet in any direction. I stand there staring off into the tree line and my brother pulls me to the other side of the porch. Jeremy, being as handy as he is, has built a giant walk-in style wooden box that occupies the left side of the porch. My brother pulls on the two wooden knobs affixed to the front doors and opens it. The inside is completely lined with foil and high powered lamps hanging at different levels from adjustable chain segments. The lamps are levitating above all different sized weed plants. Some of them look experimental, but a few of them seem to have some real promise. I wasn't expecting this at all, my interest has definitely been peaked.

"He's already has a like a pound of this shit dried out and in the freezer, there's some on the coffee table – it's not the best, but it works." My brother is gleaming with having actually surprised me. I follow him back inside the house and actually feel a little hungry. I check out the fridge and find some pasta in a Tupperware container, and decide to throw in the microwave. It's so weird to have all of the things that you need right there at your fingertips. I can't really remember the last time that I had these luxuries.

My brother rolls us up a joint from the community pot bowl that is indeed on the coffee table. It makes me think of the little wooden box, which I wish I could put right next to the clear glass bowl. I'll dig that little guy out later though. Sharing the joint with my brother feels good. I notice that Jeremy has a nice little stereo setup in the corner next to the television stand. A decent CD collection is standing next to it, mostly filled with older music from the 60's era, which is perfect right now. My brother jumps up and throws in a Doors CD, and we zone out to the music on the couch.

58. Settling

Feeling a little bit more like myself again, I decide to lay low at Jeremy's house. I'm not out looking for a job, or secluding myself indoors, but I'm just simply living. Jeremy has no problem with me squatting here, I think because he likes the company more than anything else. I feel bad for him; it's almost as if he has no friends at all. The few friends that he does seem to have aren't very good friends, and seem more like acquaintances than anything else.

Staying here has actually been fun so far. I don't really have anything to worry about, which is nice. I haven't been forced to stay clean or anything like that, but I am running dangerously low on dope, and cash for that matter. Jeremy doesn't really have any extra money that I can try to borrow from him, so I'm not really sure what I am going to do in order to score some more shit. I'm sure that I'll come up with something.

Nikki has been released from the hospital finally and is staying at a rehab facility about ten minutes away. I still haven't seen her in a couple of weeks now, but I have managed to talk to her on the phone the last few days. Jeremy actually has a phone in his house, which is also extremely convenient. You forget how great it is to be able to contact the outside world from within your own home. I can also get in touch with my brother very quickly now, and vice versa. Things are slowly starting to look up. He did the right thing by forcing me out of the apartment. I needed a change. I needed to get out of there, and it was never going to happen without some much needed assistance. This is definitely a safer environment for me to be in.

The dog has taken a particular liking to me. I think just because I seem to be as lazy as she is sometimes. We huddle up on the couch together and make fun of daytime talk shows when nobody else is around. She's a cool dog, because she's very calm and doesn't nag at you for stupid shit. She just wants to chill like everyone else. And eat, piss, shit, and sleep. That's it though – that's her list.

We have been feeding weed stems to the chinchilla. The furry little gray thing loves them. We try to give him the longest ones that we can find; sometimes they're like 18 inches long. He goes wild as he grasps his little paws around the stem and pulls in through the bars of the cage. Perched up in the air on a fake tree stump, he chews on them until they disappear completely. Then he sleeps for what seems like ever, and we do it all over again. He's been a lot of fun to play with.

We have created a small mountain of twelve pack boxes and empty bottles in the corner of the kitchen. I am trying to save up as many bottles as I can in order to build up some money for dope. I realize that they won't amount to barely anything, but for some reason I find it comforting to have them as another source. There is also a large jar of change in the closet of my room that I have had my eyes on. It doesn't seem right to steal from Jeremy, but I might not have a choice. There is a possibility that he has forgotten about its existence completely, which would make me feel better, but I can't be certain just yet. I'm waiting to see if he ever acknowledges it in any way before ultimately turning it into dope as well. I would guess that there is about 50 bucks worth of change in that jar, which would really come in handy. I might end up lifting some clothes from the local mall here. I haven't done that in so long though, and really don't want to risk getting caught if I don't have to. I need to find a safer place to steal from; sometimes it sucks living in the middle of nowhere.

My brother has been stopping in more frequently and staying on most nights for a few hours each time. He seems happier that I'm here and under some supervision, at least in the evening. He brought me a stack of rock climbing magazines that have still been getting delivered to my mom's house from an old subscription that was supposed to run out two years ago. For some reason they just keep sending them to me, and according to everyone they never send a bill. I have a stack of these now sitting on the coffee table; I look at them for hours on end whenever I'm bored. Sometimes I can't look at them though, because they make me a little depressed. Flipping through the pages I am reminded of all the things that I wouldn't even be capable of doing right now even if I wanted to. Simple movements that I used to execute on a daily basis would literally be impossible for me to perform given my current physical state. My body has been abused, and protests just about everything that would require any kind of strength. I am also reminded of the old life that I threw away so quickly and easily. I had a wonderful group of friends that have all but disappeared and moved on, not that I really blame them, but I really do miss them whenever I think about how things used to be. We were all like this weird little family all equipped with unique little roles that glued the entire mess together. It was beautiful at times. It was horrible at times. Regardless, we were all there for each other no matter what; at least that was the idea. I guess when push really comes to shove that wasn't exactly the case. I just wish sometimes that I could get things back to that time, I miss it so much. Even if I was able to change everything right now, it would never get back there. People have moved on. They've "grown up" and started to conform to "real life". It just isn't possible for it to ever be the same, so I need to stop thinking about it I guess.

A somewhat full kitchen has also been really cool. Jeremy actually has pots and pans to cook with. I am making a minestrone soup today, and for some reason I'm very excited about it. Maybe just because it's something that I haven't done in years - I have no idea. I am nonetheless very proud of it though, and can't wait for it to get done. The entire house smells like soup, which is also really cool. The small things in life are starting to make my happy. A rehab counselor would have a field day with me right now, throwing out all sorts of technical theories that they learned back in their psych classes. It would be amusing to witness actually; I wish I could get a counselor to show up here at the house just to have some mental fun with them. Halfway through the session I would seem really intent on what they were saying and pull out a needle to shoot up with right in front of them. For some reason the idea of this makes me laugh hysterically, and the dog just lifts her head to stare at me in confusion.

59. Thanksgiving

Today is thanksgiving. The holidays have been especially weird for me the last couple years. Christmas has always been at my grandparent's house. Everyone congregates there every year to open presents. My family is relatively small, so that's why it all works out this way. Last year was strange because of everything that is going on. Everyone knows about my addiction, and that I can't be trusted with cash or any other valuable merchandise for that matter. The entire event is tension filled from the minute I walk in the front door. Heroin has become that subject that people are very careful about in front of me. I'm always seen as the fragile black sheep that needs to be handled with kid gloves. It makes for a very weird day. Weird enough that it warrants smoking half a pack immediately after leaving. Needless to say the holidays themselves are always a bit stressful now, and I never look forward to them.

This year a unanimous decision has been made that I do not attend. At first there was some confusion with setting up rides, but then I think that the motivation seemed to come from other places. I gladly agreed with staying away, not having to deal with it at all was much easier for me. The verdict was set that I was going to stay here, and ironically Jeremy had nothing to do for Thanksgiving either, so we were just going to hang out and smoke all day long. That's exactly what we did.

The day started like any other day, but Jeremy was home and wasn't going to work, obviously. This was strange for me though, because he pretty much always worked. Even most weekends he'd work all day long stacking up as much extra cash as he could, which I also never understood as Jeremy never really bought anything. His truck was an old piece of shit which he clearly didn't owe any money on any more. Other than the house expenses and some occasional food he literally spends no money at all on anything. He doesn't even pay for gas, because he comes and goes every day with the flooring van, which he has a permanent company credit card for. I have no clue what he does with all of his money. I really wish that I could find a stack that he had forgotten about, but I have a feeling that he's been pretty careful with leaving cash lying around the house. He probably doesn't think that I notice, but I do. I don't blame him, if I was letting someone like myself stay at my house I'd bolt everything down to the floor.

Today is going to be cool though, I can already tell. I begin my morning by grabbing some coffee in the kitchen which Jeremy already made about an hour ago. He brewed up a gigantic pot and has everything ready to make another one as soon as this one is kicked. He's very efficient when it comes to his caffeine, which means I never have to worry about not having fresh coffee. I love how some things just work out so poetically.

After taking in as much coffee as I possibly can, I retire to my bedroom for a couple of minutes to shoot up. The day is so peaceful and quiet. The usually busy road outside has only an occasional car every fifteen minutes or so. I lean against the wall in my room next to a sleeping bag enjoying the first ten minutes of my high. Back on my feet, I make my way back out to the living room to join Jeremy in making fun of the Thanksgiving parade on TV. I still don't understand why some people like parades so much. They have always seemed pointless to me, and completely un-entertaining. I find myself drifting off somewhere else in my head whenever I see one in person or on television for that matter. Jeremy shares my dislike apparently, so I actually find a few things to laugh at as the floats drift by on the screen.

Jeremy is rolling a gigantic "Thanksgiving Joint" as he's been calling it. It looks interesting actually, he has spent about twenty-five minutes on it already, and it is quite large. He's hoping that it will last all day long. I have a feeling we'll be rolling another one by noon. It's only 10:00am and I have the entire day ahead of me for straight relaxation. This really isn't different than any other day, but for some reason in my head it feels different. It feels special. Perhaps that's just my own strange perspective of things screwing with my perception. Whatever it is, I decide to enjoy it.

Jeremy picked up some junk food yesterday on his way home from work which apparently was for the both of us. Once again – I have no complaints at all. I bring in a few bags of chips because I anticipate their immediate need, and Jeremy lights up the gargantuan joint. I have to admit – he did a good job with it. It's pulling nicely, and really hits the spot.

The afternoon rolls by slowly, and neither of us ended up doing much at all. The phone rang a few times, but we showed no interest in even seeing who called. It was a perfect day right from the beginning, much better than having to deal with strange tension filled situations with my family. I miss that things can't be the way that they used to be during the holidays, but maybe in the future there will be a way to fix that. For now this setup was perfect.

Jeremy starts pacing around the house with the phone in his hand trying to think of pizza places that would be open on Thanksgiving. He's all fired up about getting some pizza somewhere, for some reason it's the only thing that sounds good to him. I can't seem to get him interested in anything else at all. If he wanted Chinese food we'd be all set. In fact we'd be able to pick from every single Chinese food restaurant in the area, because they're all open for business like usual. They don't even see the holidays.

The phone rings again and Jeremy answers it right away, I have no idea why – I think he was being goofy. Jeremy's face lights up and he starts to chuckle a bit, which actually does sound kind of goofy. He hangs up the phone and tells me that my brother is stopping over with a bunch of leftovers from

Thanksgiving Dinner at my grandparent's house. He's going to be here in about twenty minutes. I didn't think that the day could get any better, but it was just about to.

Sure enough my brother walks in with a huge foil container that looks about four inches deep filled with all of the fixings. Turkey, mashed potatoes, stuffing, gravy, cranberry sauce, and a separate container with half of a pumpkin pie in it. I hand him "Thanksgiving Joint Number 2" with a large grin on my face, and we all grab a plate full of food.

60. Meeting

Jeremy has a not so secret stash of champagne at his house that has been here since New Years. For some unknown reason he purchased two cases of champagne for a supposed New Years Eve party that was going to occur at his house. The story goes that the location was changed at the last minute. Jeremy fails to remember that this story still doesn't explain the two almost full cases of champagne that are still here in his house. If the location was the only thing that changed one would think that he would have brought the champagne to said new location. Obviously he just got completely stood up, and it must have really sucked, because it sounds like whoever played this cruel joke on him gave him the impression that a lot of people were coming. Jeremy didn't really ever want to talk about the champagne though – he always seemed eager to get rid of it, which I was helping him do with every fifteen minutes that passed.

This is precisely what I was doing when my brother walked in the front door carrying a plastic bag full of movies. He told me that they were duplicates that he had found in his collection and was dropping them off for me. I told him to throw one in and grabbed a second glass from the kitchen along with a new bottle of champagne. Time to really start putting a dent in this stuff. My brother accepted a glass full of the bubbly and lit up a smoke. I know that my brother thinks the champagne debacle is goofy, but he has no problem partaking in its depletion.

We start watching a movie that we have both seen before, but it's been awhile. All is quiet for awhile and then Jeremy shows up from work. He quickly runs into the kitchen to grab a glass for himself. The three of us sitting in the living room drinking champagne is a funny sight. All of us so different looking, yet all holding regular glass tumblers full of pinkish colored champagne. It would make a great candid photo.

The movie keeps playing along in the background, but Jeremy is insistent on telling us this big long story of how he cut his hand today at work. He was laying down a piece of carpet in this lady's house and everything was going great. He had the utility knife in his right hand and was cutting small strips off of the carpet piece by piece in order to make it fit snugly in the corner of the room. He was hacking away at the corners of the carpet and then testing each adjustment that he made. Everything was going fine. Then everything apparently went wrong. His left hand slipped when he went to make his next cut and he ran the razor blade across the back of his fingers. He did a pretty good number on it judging by the size of the bandage that he was wearing. After spending all day waiting in the hospital he finally got his hand looked at and received no actual stitches for his cuts, but got a bunch of those butterfly sutures thrown on his hand. The whole time he told the story he was smiling as if this was some sort of accomplishment. I guess he just liked telling the story. He smiled throughout the entire story; I could tell that my brother was bored. Poor Jeremy seemed so proud as he held up his huge gauze ridden hand.

The phone rings just at the right time breaking the odd silence – It's Nikki from rehab. Jeremy hands me the phone. She's all happy to hear my voice and tells me that she is going to an AA meeting tonight at 7:30pm if I want to get a ride out and see her. It would be the only way for us to see each other because she can't have visitors in rehab. I'd have to pose as a fellow AA member – piece of cake. I wonder if I can get my brother to go with me so that it's not so boring. This might be a tough sell though. I tell her that I'll do my best to get there, but I make no promises.

Back in the living room I sit and pour us all another round of the pink bubbly. I'm trying to gauge my brother's mood to see how hard it is going to be to con him into coming with me to the meeting. To the best of my knowledge he's never been to one, I've only been to them from within rehab. I never had a problem with alcohol, so there was really no need to attend the meetings, but for some reason the rehab staff believe otherwise.

I decide to come right out with it and ask him if he'll go with me, explaining why. He gives me an odd look, but looks like he is going to give in without too much persuasion. I open another bottle of champagne and smile deeply at my brother.

"It'll be fun – we'll go drunk." I tell him laughing.

He tips his glass toward me and nods slightly.

"Fine, but you owe me." He says smiling.

We have a half hour before we need to leave for the meeting. Time to get as drunk as possible in the little time that we have. We managed to get through another full bottle before jumping in the car. My brother stayed focused on the road the whole way over, and luckily its only about ten minutes away from Jeremy's house. We arrive at the rehab center and enter though the doors right next to the facility. Elevator ride straight up to the third floor and we are seconds away from attending our first AA meeting together.

The usual degenerates seem to be in attendance tonight. A small congregation has gathered outside by the doors to get one last smoke in before braving the next thirty minutes without nicotine. In five more minutes we will be listening to our speaker of the night. I catch a glimpse of Nikki toward the rear of the room engaged in conversation with two other people who look like they volunteered their time for the meeting. She looks really good and is actually acting like a normal person. I'm shocked at first, and then immediately feel out of place within her presence. She has managed to somewhat pull herself out of this mess while I still fester somewhere right above bottom. I smile at her from across the room and she returns it happily.

It's time to take our seats. The folding metal chairs have been arranged in a very sloppy circle formation as the meeting space is too small to accommodate one large circle. My brother is to the left of me, and a stranger to my right. My brother and I are having trouble looking at each other without laughing – I'm guessing this is due to the excessive drinking that occurred before we arrived. Having him here is definitely making things more interesting. There is no chance of boredom during this meeting for either of us. He does have a nervous look on his fact though, which I attribute to this being his first time here. He'll be fine though – he always is. That's the one thing I always know about him – he doesn't need his hand held in situations like this, no matter how new they are.

The speaker starts telling us all his sad tale of alcoholism and the room is silent. All of the listeners staring at him intently and nodding along at some of his points. I have become numb to most of these tales having lived them and seen even worse on my own. I feel bad that this guy has lost his entire life and everything, but c'mon, join the fucking club. Some people find this shit helpful – I don't. It's just a big gigantic pity fest for some asshole that is willingly throwing his life away. Fuck that.

I try to steal as many looks at Nikki as I can without looking too obvious. I remember nights in her room at her parent's house, and the way that her hair would smell. It feels like those times are fifty years away, and that I'll never experience them again. This is all that's left. This is all I get.

Intermission allows us all to go outside for a smoke break. My brother and I take a walk around the building in order to speak freely about the other people in the meeting. My brother brought up a lot of funny things about certain people. This one lady was wearing a bright yellow hat that had a feather sticking up from it which my brother has found to be particularly disturbing for some reason. It was just funny to hear some of his observations. We finished our smokes and went back up to the third floor for the latter half of the meeting.

The only strange part that I wasn't quite prepared for was the serenity prayer charade. I had forgotten that we all join hands and chant the damn thing like a bunch of possessed robots. My brother looked at me in horror when he realized what was happening – this made stifling back the laughter almost impossible. Luckily it was over quickly, and we could all go back to not touching each other.

After people started to clear out I knew that my window of opportunity to see Nikki was closing, so I told my brother to wait out at the car for me. I motioned for her to come out into the hallway with me, which she did inconspicuously. Once we were out there I told her to go the women's room and that I'll be right behind her. She agreed – of course.

I enter the bathroom and lock the door behind me. Nobody else seems to be in here, so we'll be all set. I find her in the last stall wearing nothing but her bra and panties. I throw my clothes down on the cold tiled floor and she lays down on them right away. With no speaking at all – we fuck like crazy. It's a wonder that the stalls are still standing when we finish. We ended up against everything in the bathroom. On the sink counters hitting all of the faucets. Up against the large mirrors that seem to be mounted everywhere. It was a perfect release of passion for both of us, and exactly what we needed.

She was late getting back, and started to get dressed as quickly as possible. She exited first and then gave me a signal that it was safe to leave. I ran out toward my brother's car and hopped in the passenger seat smiling at him widely. He simply shook his head, and drove us back to Jeremy's place.

61. Hurdle

E van has made a few appearances at Jeremy's place over the past week. He hasn't mentioned using again. Surprisingly I think he's actually going to stick to his word about staying away from it. I don't trust it so I keep an eye on him at all times to make sure that he isn't secretly obsessing over it. He's just about made a believer out of me. I won't be entirely convinced until more time passes, but for now he's got me. My biggest worry about Evan is finally able to take a back seat. I'm glad that I wasn't successful in ruining yet another person's life. I'm so grateful that Jeremy wants nothing to do with heroin. He draws the line at pot, and that's fine with me.

I have heard through Jeremy that Brad is not doing very well these days. He works with one of Brad's cousins on occasion. Apparently he is living at a different cousin's house and has found himself in trouble with the law quite a bit lately mainly for theft. He stole a car a few weeks ago and got arrested after a small chase throughout the city. He did a few days in jail before he was finally bailed out, and is going to face a gigantic fine for the stunt that he pulled. He is still just hanging around the house using like crazy day in and day out. I suppose in a lot of ways I'm no better than he is though. I just haven't gotten into any trouble lately, aside from that I am living the same exact life so who am I to judge.

I haven't seen Nikki since the night at the AA meeting, but at least I walked away with a very fond memory. I have been able to speak to her a few times on the phone, and I must admit that she sounds really good – convincing even. If I didn't know better I'd really think that she was going to stay clean this time. I hope that I'm wrong, but if you ask me she must have all of those counselors in rehab snowballed into believing that she's gotten better and turned a corner in her life. I hope that I'm wrong.

Hurdle

My brother is coming over in a few minutes and we are going to make the famous minestrone soup together this time. I'm really looking forward to doing it for some reason. I used to love to cook, and even considered getting into the culinary arts at one point, but after learning about all of the work that would ultimately go into making it a career, that thought quickly faded. The soup that I made a few days ago was missing a few vegetables, so my brother is bringing over those essentials today. I think that it will be fun.

My brother shows up right when he said that he would with a plastic bag in hand from the grocery store. We make our way to the kitchen and decide to get everything rolling on the soup. My brother is cutting the vegetables while I start preparing the stock. We move around the kitchen with swiftness while the stereo in the living room is cranked. It's a very peaceful time that requires no talking. We work very well together, and should probably do this more often. I'm glad I had the idea to make the soup again or else we wouldn't even be doing this.

After about twenty-five minutes or so everything is simmering in a giant pot on the stove, and the house is beginning to smell amazing. Snow flurries have started making an appearance outside, and the smell of the cooking soup is perfect. We both sit down on the couch and prepare to relax for a little bit. My brother starts rolling a joint from the communal weed bowl on the coffee table, and both of us are smiling in unison. This is another one of those little moments that I wish I could freeze and hold onto forever. I don't want it to ever end.

After an hour or so the front door opens and Jeremy walks in with a puzzled look on his face. He's holding a letter in one hand, and a torn open envelope in the other.

"I'm losing my house." Jeremy utters in our general direction.

"How so?" I ask staring at him in shock.

"A hotel company has purchased all of this land, including the land that the house is on. They are offering to buy me out so that they can knock the house down and construct a hotel right here!" He replies in a frustrated tone.

"By the looks of it I don't even really have a choice."

"What's the time frame?" I ask immediately thinking about how this is going to affect everything.

"A month." Jeremy answers, this time with even more shock in his voice.

My brother is just sitting there looking back and forth between Jeremy and myself. I try to think of something comforting to say, but I come up with nothing. Jeremy looks as though somebody just kicked him in the nuts. Honestly I don't blame him. He had everything he'd ever need right here in this house. The amount of land that he has is perfect, and the privacy is priceless. He's been here for about five years or so and already has a descent amount of the house paid off, according to some conversations that we have had recently. He's going to have to scramble and come up with a new living situation within the next thirty days. Jeremy isn't stupid, but he's not the brightest, most assertive person that there is. This is not going to be an easy task for him to pull off, and that's assuming that he tackles it when he's of sound mind, which he clearly is not at the moment. The first thing that I think about is the weed shed that he built on the back porch. I know that wouldn't really be an immediate concern for most people, but I find an immense sadness in thinking of that little shed being destroyed. They are forcing him to give up so many things. They are forcing him to change his entire life in just a mere thirty days. I'd be just as pissed as he is right now, perhaps even more so.

"Listen man, if there's anything that either of us can do to help make sure that you let me know. It's the least that I can do and I'm more than happy to help in any way that I can." I say to Jeremy with nothing but sincerity.

Hurdle

He acknowledges my offering and says "thanks" in a voice that is only mildly louder than a whisper. He makes his way through the living room and heads straight to his room. I have a feeling that he'll be in there for awhile – poor bastard. My brother is looking at me with a puzzled look now too.

"Where are you going to go? Not back to the apartment. Right?" He asks me – not wanting to hear my answer.

"Well it's the only place that I can go right now, unless I think of something else in the meantime. I don't really have a choice." I answer quickly, and then head out to the kitchen to check on the soup. My brother follows me slowly and the entire atmosphere of the day has changed in an instant. The peacefulness that was once floating through the air with such tenacity has been replaced with fear of the unknown. Sadness has seeped into the house as if a black cloud has completely covered the ceiling in every room. I knew that I wanted to freeze that moment of us on the couch for a reason.

62. Plans

Jeremy is really still unhappy with the hotel situation. A few days have passed and his spirits don't seem to be getting any better. I doubt that mine would either if I was in his position, but it's just weird to see Jeremy down. He's usually so happy, sometimes even annoyingly so. Being around him now is uncomfortable simply for that reason. When somebody acts completely out of character than what you are used to it tends to make things a bit awkward. I can't think of anything that I can do to help him, and I can barely think of how I am going to handle my own situation. I'm going to miss staying here though; it was a very interesting period of time.

As I look back on the last couple of weeks I find myself smiling at each little memory. Jeremy laughing hysterically and dropping pizza all over the floor. My brother hanging out with one of his friends and playing drinking games with us all night. There were lots of funny things that happened that night. I don't remember the last time that I laughed so hard my stomach hurt – but it did that night. I'm going to miss the freedom that we all have here. Everyone is just able to be themselves with no judgment, and somehow in the end it all works out. A configuration like this one happens only once in a lifetime, and I realize that I'll never experience it again. That is the root of my sadness right now. Not knowing where I am going to go or what I am going to do is the least of my worries, because I know that I'll always find my way. Leaving this all behind is the problem, and I want us all to have as much fun as we possibly can before it's time to go. I owe my brother so much for dragging me here and making all of this happen in the first place. It was exactly what I needed, and at exactly the right time.

I have started throwing around the idea of getting another job, but I am still not sold on it. I am pissed that I managed to screw up the stocking job at the store – it was perfect. They obviously won't even look at me if I tried to get it back, so the only other option is to get that position at yet another grocery store in the area. The problem with that is that all of these stores are so different from each other in the way that they are run. If I ever have to go back to a place that resembles my first grocery store career I'll never be able to make it. I will blow my head off during the very first shift out of sheer desperation and boredom. I can't go back to another place like that ever again. For the time being I am going to remain unemployed, but I am at least toying with the idea of seeking employment again in the future – if I can think of something to do that won't kill me in the process. Eventually I'll figure out something I'm sure.

As far as a living situation, I might not have a choice but to return to the apartment with Nikki. I assume that she is on her way back there, although I haven't heard from her in a couple of days. Rehab was supposed to end for her soon, I figured that she'd call me when she got out, but I haven't heard from her yet. I can't see any reason why she wouldn't go back there, as the rent is already paid for another month and a half. I fear what will happen if we end up living together again. Even if she is clean right now, if I start living with her again she'll probably go right back to using, unless she has really somehow turned into another person entirely. The two of us are very destructive together – I might have to come up with another living solution. At the moment I have nothing else in mind – I've run out of places to go for the most part.

I can hear the wooden box in my room shaking underneath a pile of clothes. It's reminding me that it's time to use again. It's been about eight hours or so since my last fix, and my arms are starting to itch with anticipation. I have managed to somewhat control my heroin use over the last week and a half or so, but I am no longer in denial. I need to stop. I still can't figure out how I am going to accomplish this monumental task, but I ultimately need to find a way. I can control the frequency of my use now with more precision than ever before. I can actually wait until I can't take it anymore, and the time intervals have pretty much stuck to a strict schedule. In the past I was only able to do this for a day or so and then everything would collapse and go to shit. Now however I am doing it successfully ever day, which is affording me the ability to think clearly in between hits. It still has an incredible hold on me, the biggest hold of anything else in the entire world, but now I can see it clearer. Now I have the time to think and plot. Scheme and work up strength against it. I've found a way in, and I'm going to use it. I just need more time. My stash is getting low and I might need to make one more trip to the big city before I can work up the strength that I am going to need to beat it. I might have to call in help from Evan in order to get transportation. I don't want to do this, but I might not have a choice in the matter. If one more hit for Evan gets me what I need and pushes me one step closer to perhaps getting clean – then I'll let it happen. Sometimes you have to destroy something else in order to yield a better overall outcome. I have been shown that Evan can handle it, and it's been a long time since his last hit. I have all the confidence in the world that one more hit a month later won't force him into becoming an addict. I could be wrong, but I doubt it. Either way I might end up deeming it worth taking the chance. The next month is going to be interesting – I can feel it. It is going to be filled with impossibilities, and other hardships. Temptation will be around every corner, taunting me to do the wrong thing. I'll be constantly tested and I might constantly fail. Regardless, it's about time that I actually gave it a shot.

63. Division

Today we harvest. Jeremy has decided to get rid of all the pot that he has grown; transporting the plants would be too difficult – especially seeing as how he still has no idea where he is going. The weed shed that Jeremy constructed on the back porch is going to need some dismantling before move day as well. Sadly he is even sacrificing the mother plant that he has devoted so much time to over the past few months. It will be sad to see it all go, but because Jeremy is such a giving person, I just nailed my money solution for more dope. He's giving me half of his crop. All I have to do is help with the process of drying it out. How could I decline such an offer?

My brother is going to come over and give me a hand as well, not to mention that he has already found us a buyer for the product. I should have a little under a pound of pretty descent stuff by the time all is said and done. My brother has already found a buyer who'll take the entire thing off of our hands for about $3,500. This is going to be some of the easiest cash I have ever made. We haven't told Jeremy about our hook up, because he'd be a little upset that we were already able to turn it into cash. Instead we are just going to pretend that we want it for personal use. It shouldn't really matter as I probably won't see Jeremy for awhile after this month is over. There's no telling where I am going to end up, and I have a feeling that he's going to grab a small apartment somewhere for the time being. Ultimately he wants to get another house, but he wants it to be very similar in nature to this one. Location, land, and privacy are all key components to what he is looking for, and that really narrows down the selection. At least he seems to be dealing the reality of it all a lot better now that a few days have passed. He's even seeing it as a blessing in disguise because there are a handful of repairs on this place that he hasn't had time to deal with yet. The atmosphere in the house today is much less glum than it has been.

Jeremy walks out to the living room with the mother plant hanging from a broom handle. The buds are large and measure about eight inches long. It's sticky and very pungent in smell. Thankfully the house is getting leveled, because this smell would be here for an eternity. It's sad to see the mother in such a compromising position, but it's going to hook me up with cash so I quickly get over it. Jeremy seems to be taking it very well also, he's proud of the product that he has been able to create. It's ironic that once his perfection was attained, he was forced to destroy it. He's confident that he can recreate the formula in the future, however.

Two scales are out on the coffee table and a stack of clear plastic baggies rest in between them – all different shapes and sizes. Jeremy has some people that he works with that buy from him, so he starts preparing their bags right away to get the small stuff done and weighed out. I can tell that he hates having to break buds in half in order to weigh things out properly. Hesitation shakes through his hands as he carefully turns a six inch bud into two separate pieces. If it was up to him everyone would buy an amount that required no alteration of the buds – but that's not really reality, unless of course you are the buyer that my brother found. We lucked out on that one.

I start weighing out my share and bagging up things as necessary. Just for effect I weigh out one ounce bags and keep the entire load separate. This way Jeremy can't suspect that I have already found someone to punt the entire pound to. I'd feel bad hurting his feelings, so who cares? I'll just mix it all together later. Jeremy keeps working along not noticing anything weird about what I am doing – perfect. Just then my brother walks in and takes a seat on the floor on the opposite side of the coffee table.

"I'm rolling guys." He announces and takes a small bud from the pile. He crumbles it up on the table in front of him with concentration and precision. You would think that he was decorating a cake with the fragility in which he handles the weed. It's funny how serious he takes things sometimes. It's like he puts his heart and soul into every little thing that he does. It's a quality that I sometimes wish I had.

My brother didn't roll very well, but he knew this already. He considered each joint another chance toward perfection. For his consideration we all dealt with whatever sloppy shape he managed to roll up. In the long run it never really mattered anyways, a joint is a joint for the most part. It was kind of funny though when you thought about it. Eventually he'll master his technique I'm sure. Today's joint actually didn't come out that bad. He hands it to me for the honorable lighting ceremony. It burns nice right from the first hit. I flash him an approving look as I pass it to Jeremy. A smirk comes to life on his face – he's proud of his work.

Jeremy is almost done weighing and bagging his share of the load and decides to order a pizza. This is common behavior for him, he's too impatient to have a discussion about food, so instead he just bites the bullet and gets a pizza that he knows everyone will like. Of course we never complain.

While waiting for the pizza to arrive I sit on the couch thinking about the more immediate future. Scoring dope is my number one priority for right now, I need to call Evan in a few hours and setup transportation for tomorrow. I have only two hits left in the wooden box, which is cutting it very close. I could always settle for something around here, but it's just not the same. It's actually worth the trip to get the stuff I'm used to.

My brother snaps me out of my daze when he holds up all of the baggies in his hands indicating that it's all done. I smile in approval again, and he fills up his backpack with the load.

64. Stash

Everything is lined up as planned. My brother punted off the weed and scored exactly what he said he would. He took a grand leaving me with $2500 to do what I will with. He was against me having cash, but I convinced him that things were going to change and that he needed to trust me on this one. With great reluctance he handed it over and walked away, looking devastated that he had given in to me. I'm going to do everything I can to prove to him it was the right move to make. I just need a little more time.

Evan has agreed to let me use his car, and seemed indifferent about using. He wasn't uninterested, but he wasn't ecstatic either. He may have just been trying to hide his enthusiasm from me. I'm glad that he wasn't jumping out of skin to use, but I'm not sure if I trust his acting. I'll have a better idea about where things stand tonight. Evan's going to hang out here while I make the trip – he should be here any minute.

I have everything that I need for the trip ready to go when he walks in the front door. He tosses me his keys and I'm out within thirty seconds. Time to get serious. It's been awhile since I came out here, and my last trip was horrid. Not going out here as much as I used to, I have to remember to keep my head and not mess up. It's not that hard, but sometimes I have to remind myself to stay in the zone. It's not safe out here, even if it appears to be. One false step can land me in a world of shit – as I have already found out many times before. Get in, get out – that's what I'm here to do.

The city is like a giant network of veins that get fed everyday from the enormous syringe which emerges from the sky. The needle delivers a daily dose of shit that litters the streets with crime. Until that needle is destroyed this place will always be a cesspool. An endless sea of work for local law enforcement. A bottomless pit of junkies with nowhere else to go. Today – I'm just a visitor.

The tattered house is beginning to look a bit more tattered. Some of the shudders have fallen off leaving behind the unpainted rectangle of space next to their respective windows. The chain link fence that surrounds the front yard is also starting to show some wear. It looks as though a car may have even hit one corner of it causing the metal to mold together in a giant tangled mass. I don't miss coming here. Walking the path to the front door always made me feel a bit uneasy. I just have to stay cool today as I take the journey through the gate at the edge of the sidewalk. Eyes straight and one hand on the cash.

The guy at the window recognizes me this time. He smiles at me with disbelief when I tell him how much I want. Then I produce the stack of twenties on the small shelf. He gets to work counting out packets. The only downside to getting a descent quantity is the length of time it takes to be sorted out and finally plopped down on the little shelf in front of me. Standing here creates a feeling of vulnerability that is hard to explain. Imagine that you are completely naked on a stage in the largest auditorium you can think of. Everyone is there staring at you, and there is complete and utter silence. Then – just when you think that there is no possible way things could get any worse – A large man comes up behind you and starts railing you in the ass. You look up to see everyone still staring at you. Silence still blaring throughout the building. That's about how vulnerable I feel right now.

Finally the process is done and the dope is there in front of me. $2000 worth – should last me a couple of weeks at least. I pocket the stuff quickly and head back out toward the street, leaving faded foot prints in the light snow that has covered the ground. Evan's car is great in the snow so I have nothing to worry about as far as the weather is concerned. I make my way back up the street toward the car – get in and lock the doors. Big exhale – I'm on my way out of here.

Driving by the diner near the highway has never been the same. I always look at it as I coast by. A nervous lump develops in my stomach every time. I'll never be able to go in there again, which saddens me, perhaps when I'm like fifty I'll be able to get away with it. Thanks a lot Brad. Getting away from him was one of the best things that I ever did. It didn't prevent me from being homeless and bottoming out so many times, but I fear that worse things would have happened if we stuck together. Brad is bad news all around. I'm surprised he's even still alive.

The highway is dead today on the way home – which is really nice considering my return trip last time. I'm also of sound mind which plays a key role in all of that. Last time I was sweating profusely and fighting to keep my hands on the wheel. That was a bad time for me. I am much more peaceful today though. One of my favorite tapes is cranking along in Evan's car as I fly down the two lane road. I feel really good for the most part. I left myself a good chunk of money to live on for the next month or so, food won't be a problem. Neither will alcohol or smokes for that matter, which reminds me to stop at the package store before I get to Jeremy's place.

I load up on some beer that I know everyone likes and grab a few bottles of vodka to get the job done quicker and with better results. I tell the guy at the counter to throw in a carton of smokes, and I'm all stocked up for awhile. It feels really good. Back out in the car I make my way a few more miles to Jeremy's house. He's still not home from work yet – so Evan and I can get high in the living room. Even though Jeremy doesn't have a problem with it, I still don't like my shit around anyone who isn't directly involved. It's weird enough to openly do it with Evan, and he's actually using at the time. It's just something that I still can't seem to get my head around.

Stash

Evan is flipping through the channels when I walk in the house. He looks up smiling, and kills the TV. I go to my room to retrieve the box and Evan flips some Pink Floyd on the stereo. I hear it come on from my room and immediately can't wait to get high. Some music just puts you right in the mood for mind alteration experiences. The fact that they were able to capture that essence in sound alone is amazing. The next few hours are going to be magical for me, and being in such a relaxed state will definitely help. I can hear my pulse slowly pumping in my ears as I open the small box and drop all of the packets inside. I walk out to the living room to find Evan sitting on the couch with his shirt off – he's looking forward to this too.

65. Thoughts

The music is pulsing throughout the living room. It's all that I can hear as I sit slumped into the corner of the couch. Thoughts swirl around in my head slowly and bleed into each other as the music continues on. Evan is in a similar state, but seems to be awake with his eyes wide open. I notice that he's nodding along to the sound emitting from the speakers. It's very quiet in the house otherwise. Jeremy's dog is lying on the couch in between the two of us sleeping away. She's all sprawled out on her back – a mass of golden fur and paws everywhere.

Suddenly Kristen's face enters my head, a perfect outline of blond hair accompanied by those gleaming white teeth. I miss her greatly, and should really try to get in touch with her. I've stayed away ever since the overdose episode at her house. My mother has kept in touch with her here and there and gives me updates whenever I talk to her. I am avoiding the shame that I will feel the first time I see her again. It was wrong of me to impose on her the way that I did, and I will forever feel remorseful. I miss her company, and the things that we used to do together. I miss all of the cute little things that she used to do – like putting in a great CD whenever I showed up, or whipping up a great batch of coffee. I think I miss her scent the most though. The way that she would smell, at any given time, was enough to bring me to my knees. If I could bottle up her scent and carry it with me always – I would.

Enough about Kristen – the more I think about her the more depressed I get. I have to get her off of my mind. Nikki is out in the world somewhere – I know it. I still haven't heard from her, which is a little bit odd, but at the same time she can be a bit flighty. I am curious as to where she is and how she is doing. Last I knew we were still together so I'm not sure what's going on exactly. My brother hasn't run into her or else he surely would have given me an update. It's as if she has completely disappeared. I'm going to have my brother swing by the apartment to see if she is there, or if there is any sign of life in it for that matter. It wouldn't surprise me to find out that she has gone off in a completely separate direction. Not much would surprise me at this point.

Evan struggles to get to his feet and heads toward the kitchen. I stay glued in my spot, not feeling the need for any immediate movement. He returns with a bag of chips that I picked up at the liquor store. I don't even know why I ended up getting them, they must have looked good at the time – right now I think I'd die if I ate one. I reach out toward the coffee table and retrieve my pack of smokes. That's the only thing that sounds good to me at the moment. Evan is sitting on the couch in a strange position chomping away at the bag of chips. It's all I can do to prevent myself from laughing hysterically. If only I could take a picture of him right now to show him later. I've never seen anyone sit the way that he is. Some of the smallest things in the world are so funny to me sometimes. It doesn't make any sense.

The dog is still passed out in the same position despite Evan's movements. She could sleep through the demolition of the house when the time comes. Lazy old dog – she's cool shit. The phone rings, and luckily it is sitting on the coffee table or else answering it would never have been entertained. I pick it up slowly and check the caller ID. It's a number that I don't recognize at all – which makes me very leery of picking up. I hit the talk button and say hello in a somewhat strange voice just in case. It's Nikki. Apparently she is staying at a half-way house a few blocks away from rehab. I've been there before to see certain people, but not to actively live there. It was recommended that she not be out in the world completely on her own yet, especially with the wonderful progress that she has displayed while in rehab. At the half-way house she is some sort of counselor type person in charge of helping others who are still really messed up in their addictions. She is planning on being there for another two weeks or so. I tell her about Jeremy's and what is happening to his house. She's surprised, but doesn't really seem that concerned about it. She acts as though she has moved on in some monumental way. I'm not sure if I particularly like this version of Nikki. I can tell that she has gobbled up a lot of the psychobabble that gets thrown around in rehab. They have managed to keep her away from her drug for the time being, but have changed her completely in the process. In my opinion that's just as bad, and precisely my biggest issue with getting clean. I don't want to change who I am at all, except for the addiction itself. I don't think that I am even capable of this drastic change though, and I never thought that Nikki was. I guess I was wrong there. We hang up and I feel like getting high again – but I don't.

Evan is still in the same funny position on the couch and he's still eating chips. This time I can't take it anymore and I start laughing my ass off. He turns his head slowly in my direction with a confused look on his face, still chewing away. I laugh even harder. Other than his blank stare, he has no other reaction to my laughter. I really wish that we could generate a print out of what is going on in his head right now, I bet that's even funnier than what I am laughing at. I gasp for breath in between laughing fits and Evan just turns his head back toward the empty television screen. I light another smoke and sink back into the couch behind me.

According to my calculations I have about three weeks left until this house is going to be leveled by massive amounts of heavy machinery. Giant yellow bulldozers will drive down the long driveway and tear right through the front door. The living room will collapse in on itself first and be pushed through the kitchen. The bedrooms will be annihilated and bathroom parts will fall into the mix of shattered wood and broken sheetrock. My plan right now is to return to the apartment in the hopes that Nikki is going to move on and not want to return. She didn't mention going back on the phone, and with the giant corner she has seemingly turned in her life she might see it as a reminder of her addiction. This mentality will guarantee that she'll stay away. The only thing worse than the drug an addict is addicted to is the plan that they then obsess over to stay away from said drug. She's on a path to becoming the world's biggest protestor of drugs – created by the state. I'll use that to my advantage for as long as I can.

66. Heist

It's 10:00am the next morning and I am startled by a knock at the door. This can't be good. This doesn't happen here. Jeremy is at work and my brother has a key. Evan would have called first I'm sure, and there really isn't anybody else who even knows that I'm here. Nikki does, but she's off in her own little world, I doubt that she put any effort into finding a way to get to me.

I tiptoe through the living room and creep up to one of the windows on the side of the front door. Peeking through the blinds I can see the outline a man standing on the front steps. It doesn't register right away who I'm looking at. Loose jeans and a black non-descript hoodie two sizes too large impatiently rocking back and forth on the step. Then it hits me – It's Brad. Fuck. This is not good at all. I argue with myself for a few moments before I reach over and open the door. I never should have allowed myself to do so.

Brad is looking at me like he's never met me before, and then he smiles widely while walking into the living room.

"I've got the best score for us – you aren't going to believe this." He says to me bursting with excitement.

"No how have you been? Just cut right to the chase?" I sneer back at him.

"C'mon man, I've missed hanging out, and besides you are the one that ran out on me remember? I woke up and you were gone – half the shit was gone – but I've gotten over it. You have got to hear me out on this one though – it's perfect." He says still smiling like a fool.

"Fine – I'm listening."

Brad goes on to tell me his grand scheme. He's working at a uniform plant right now, when he goes to work that is, and he's been privy to some information about a certain family that is currently out of town. He overheard a conversation that he wasn't supposed to between one of his co-workers and his supervisor. Apparently there is a pretty well off family who is friends with his supervisor that are hitting the road for a couple of weeks. They have a gigantic house at the end of a woodsy road on the nice, safe side of town. Brad got all of the details as to when there isn't going to be anyone there watching over it. The great thing about his plan is that there is no way to connect him to the crime. He'll be completely dissociated from it, as will I if I agree to join him. He claims that it will end up being the perfect crime. The house has got to be loaded with priceless items such as jewelry and other fine art pieces. Brad is expecting to score a lot of cash with this one. He's done this shit in the past and even gotten busted for it a few times. It's not good to have breaking and entering charges on your record; he has to be really careful. Another charge would surely land him in jail for a period of time.

His plan is that we go there tonight. His supervisor has been assigned house duty for the next two weeks, but he won't be there tonight, or tomorrow night for that matter. That fact makes the crime even more perfect, because time will pass before anybody even knows that it has happened. I agree to the plan with some reluctance, because I am for some reason unable to say no when it comes to certain things. I can't bring myself to feel bad about it. Stealing from someone who has an endless supply of disposable income seems very justifiable to me. I'm sure that they have some sort of house insurance anyways that will just replace all of these pointless items for them. Then everyone can calm down and get their rest once again. I'm all for ripping these fuckers off.

Brad tries to spark up conversation with me, but I'm not interested. Things have changed since before. I've hardened on some level and can't tolerate Brad's ramblings anymore. I see right through his words and find myself becoming annoyed with just about everything he says. He doesn't know shit, which is why he always fucks everything up and gets busted in the end. This is not going to be some grand reunion – our time together is over, and that's exactly how it is going to remain.

In the middle of a sentence I get up off the couch and head toward my bedroom.

"Hey, where you going?" Brad asks flustered.

"To get some dope to shut your ass up, you're driving me nuts. I can't take it anymore." I answer surprised at how forward I am.

Brad doesn't even respond. I knew that I could bribe him into silence. He's so powerless over heroin. He's like an obedient lap dog as soon as you pull it out or mention its coming. I set the wooden box down in front of him and motion him to get to it. He opens it up and his eyes swell up to the size of melons. He's astonished at the amount of dope just sitting there ready to go. He chuckles a few times and pulls out what he needs to hook himself up with. I grab another coffee and sit on the other side of the couch waiting for him to get done. Brad shoots it and looks at me smiling like I'm a god for having such wonderful shit on hand. I make a face at him and slide the box across the coffee table. I want this afternoon to go by as fast as possible. I give myself a healthy dose praying for coma-like sleep – and that's exactly what I get.

I wake up and it's dark out already. Brad is sitting on the couch watching Oprah of all fucking things. I can't even stand the sound of that bitch's voice – it must have been what woke me up.

"Turn that shit off." I shout at Brad who jumps at the sound of my voice. What a loser. I decide to go take a shower in order to get ready for the big heist. While in the shower I start to think about the house we are going to be busting into. I wonder if they have a dog. Or at least a cat, but that wouldn't really matter. I suppose it wouldn't matter if they had a dog either – as long as it's a nice dog. They have kids though so most likely the dog is nice. I don't really know a lot of suburban families with trained killer pit-bulls guarding their overpriced houses. It is something to consider though. I wonder if the house has an alarm. I think that a lot of people are doing that alarm shit now; I'll have to ask Brad if he knows anything about that. He must under the impression that they don't though; otherwise I'd like to think that he wouldn't be entertaining this plan. I can't think of any other deterring factors though except for those two things. An alarm would surely screw us, a dog we could probably handle. I'm feeling pretty good about the whole thing.

Brad seems to be emerging from the couch when I come out of my room. I grab the wooden box and toss any paraphernalia that has made its way onto the table back inside. Brad looks at me funny as I do this, obviously wondering why I am bothering to pick it all up. I just ignore him and bring it back into my room, stashing it in the closet beneath a pile of clothes. I come back out and Brad is heading toward the door – looks like it's time to go.

We hop into the car that Brad showed up in. I'm not sure if it's his or not, nor do I care. I don't even bother talking during the ride across town to the desolate road with the giant house on it. We stop at a small park right at the beginning of the road so that we can stash the vehicle. Just in case something happens, at least the car will be safe. On foot we start walking down the road. There are houses every two hundred feet or so, spread far apart from each other. Large yards are attached to each lot, and the houses are set way back from the road. Some of them you can't even see between the trees that line the driveways with such density. There's no way that we'll be spotted on our journey to the vacant monstrosity.

After about ten minutes of walking through the brisk cold air the enormous brown house comes into view. An elaborate circular window hovers about the front door exposing a spiraled staircase leading to the second floor. A magnificent chandelier hangs in view above the staircase. There must be some good things in there to loot. I follow Brad toward the rear of the house which is equipped with a giant deck and built in hot tub. French doors line one wall of the deck leading into the kitchen and dining area of the house. Brad heads for the door. He pulls out a cordless drill and starts drilling right through the lock. So far I see no sign of pets outside the house. Other than the two of us and the noise of the drill – there are no other sounds to be heard. After about two minutes Brad has the door opened and he's motioning me inside after him.

The kitchen is huge, larger than any normal person would ever dream of needing. The counters are a dark red marble and the island in the middle matches it. There's a small flat screen television installed in the wall underneath one of the many cabinets. The floors are all hardwood and look as though they have never been walked on before. Even with just the moonlight shining in through the glass doors behind us, the floor gives off a shine that is almost blinding. I don't even want to see the rest of the house. Brad heads straight for the spiraled staircase and I follow behind him in awe.

The master bedroom is even more of a sight to behold. It seems as though it is the entire footprint of the house in size – a room that never seems to end in any direction. A full couch and love seat setup is on one side of the room surrounding a giant wall mounted flat screen television. It's a second living room, perhaps nicer than the one downstairs actually. A full bar is in another corner of the elaborate room. Windows are everywhere and come right down to the floor where they meet the plush white carpet. A California king bed is plopped into the center of the other half of the room. More French doors on one side of the bed seem to lead out to a balcony of sorts which faces the woods behind the house. Looking out the doors is when I notice the

Heist

large barn type shed a hundred feet away from the house. The yard is very large and has a gigantic rock formation in the middle of it. A small fountain spurts from the center of the rocks and forms a stream which circles the entire formation. My staring is jolted when we hear the phone ring echoing throughout the empty house. Both Brad and I jump and then start laughing at each other. It's just the phone. Brad continues pawing through the contents of the jewelry box which he has emptied out on the bed. A small mountain of gold and jewels has formed in front of Brad's hands. He yanks a pillow case off of one of their designer pillows and starts filling it up. I just sit on the bed and stare around the room, noticing every little detail that has been put into making this house as perfect as possible. The molding that runs around the edge of the ceiling has been chosen with careful consideration. The shape of the bed frame matches the rest of the furniture on purpose. Lots of time and money has been put into every little thing that exists here. It's just another addiction that happens to be acceptable.

A large crashing sound makes its way up the staircase and into the master bedroom. Brad and I look up at each other in an instant. At first I'm frozen to the bed not understanding what is happening. The next moment I am on the balcony outside and climbing down the side of it as fast as I can. I'm not sure where Brad went, but he's about to be fucked I'm sure. The cops are here. The hardwood floors downstairs seemed to be flooded with footsteps immediately following the large bang of the kicked in door. Shouting voices screaming "police". There must have been a fucking alarm. I didn't even think about it again on the way over, or when were inside. It must have been silent. There's no other way that they could have known we were there. At least they don't know how many of us were inside, and nobody has made it to the backyard yet, so I still have a chance. I just have to get behind the shed.

I'm hanging from the floor of the balcony for about two seconds before I let go and hope I land ok. The ground hits me hard and knocks the wind out of me. The snow that has accumulated is glazed over with ice and didn't do much to dampen my fall. I struggle to my feet and look toward the shed. That's the first time that I hear the dogs. Fuck. I set off running as fast as I can while supporting my ankle that is killing me from the fall. I make it halfway to the shed before three German Shepherds launch themselves at my back and take me down. Both arms pinned in their mouths and one on my leg – I am pinned in the snow not able to move away from their grip. Three cops are cuffing me a minute later as the dogs snarl in my direction while they sit there obediently next to their masters. I see Brad being pushed into a police car by two other cops as I'm escorted to my free ride to the station. They stuff me into the small space in a similar manner, and just like that the giant house full of useless shit is safe again.

67. Resistance

It's the same old shit at the station. Brad and I are split up during processing, and I have a feeling that it's going to stay that way. The cops are giving us shit the whole time and laughing at us for apparently being stupid. There was indeed a silent alarm on the house. The goddamn alarm panel is in plain view in the living room, and upstairs in the hallway. Since we went in through the back of the house and used the main staircase we didn't see either of them. Going straight to the master bedroom was our biggest mistake. One swift run through the living room would have given the alarm away and we could have gotten out of there in plenty of time. I never should have answered the door this morning when I realized it was Brad standing there. I should have just pretended that I wasn't there, if the situation ever presents itself again that's exactly what I am going to do. I have no problem telling him that at this point either. Granted I shouldn't have even agreed to do it in the first place, but if he didn't bring it all to my attention I would never be in this position right now.

The processing is done and my bail is set to $1200. Surprisingly I might even be able to come up with it this time. Between the left over cash that I have from the pot sale and my brother's grand I might be able to get out of here tonight. I make my only phone call to my brother. He doesn't seem happy about having to use his grand, but he agrees after a minute or so and says he'll be right out to get me. This irritates the arresting officers – they don't want to see me to go.

Brad on the other hand is being held without bail due to his record. I knew that was going to bite him in the ass one day. I'm glad, because he's not going to be able to follow me out of here, which I'm sure he'd do if he could. They throw Brad in a cell and hand me my manila envelope of personal items that they took off of me during processing. I really didn't have anything on me, so the need for the envelope was nil, but they can't break protocol.

My brother shows up and gives one of the officers a dirty look before we leave. The cop shouts something unintelligible at him as we leave, but he just ignores him and keeps walking. I'm sure that pissed the officer off even more. My brother hates cops, probably even more than I do, which is surprising to me. He hasn't really had that many run-ins with them, but apparently the ones he's had have been enough to mold his perception. You can only get away with so much when it comes to my brother before he writes you off as useless and sees right through the bullshit you're spinning. It's another great quality that he has; I can gauge things better when he's around, judging by his reactions. It's a good balance.

He drives us back to Jeremy's and starts giving me shit for hanging out with Brad. I explain to him what happened, and he starts to come around a little bit. I can tell that he's trying to not blow up at me about using, which I appreciate, but at the same time I can see where I deserve it. If I was in his shoes I would have already lost it. We arrive at Jeremy's and my brother tells me that he can't stay tonight – he has some shit to do. I say goodbye and walk inside.

Jeremy is sitting on the couch watching mindless TV. He's the only one here who actually uses that damn thing. Sometimes it annoys me because he'll laugh uncontrollably at things that I don't find to be funny. I try to block it out as much as I can, but I just don't understand the mentality behind it. If something is legitimately funny – fine laugh your ass off – but most of it is just regurgitated garbage. I don't get it.

I head to my room. Music is playing in my head as I walk down the hallway. I need to get high. I need to shut my mind off and get some sleep. I'm supposed to show up in court tomorrow, but I'm not going to go. I can't go to jail right now. I can't afford a giant fine right now even if I'm able to evade a jail sentence. I can't go to rehab right now – I'll never make it. I need this time for myself in order to get better. I need to have the power to carry out this plan without something on the outside fucking it up. Every week something has to come and interfere in my life. It can't happen that way anymore. I need to take matters into my own hands. I'm going to lay low and fly under the radar for as long as I can until I am ready to take it all head on. I have enough dope to bring me forward to the next step. Nobody can trace me back to Jeremy's house, so I'll be safe here. Brad won't give me up if he's asked either, I know that. Brad would never rat somebody out – even if he didn't like the person. He's against it on principle, a priceless quality to possess.

I am going to have to spend as much time here as possible for the next couple of weeks, which should be easy enough to do. I can get whatever I need from the outside world through my brother, and I already have the essentials here anyway hidden away in the little wooden box. I can do this. I am nervous about what will ultimately come of the breaking and entering charge, especially with skipping out on court, but it can't be worse than missing a court date for possession which I've already dealt with in the past.

I setup shop on the corner of my mattress so that I can get high and drift off to sleep. The moonlight is making its way into the window and lighting up the wooden box ever so slightly. It reminds me of the hardwood floors in that house, but only if they had been used and weathered over time. That's what the box looks like at least. Dull and unpolished. Used and abused even. It just adds to its overall character. I stroke the top of the box lightly with my fingertips before I succumb to its power and flip it open.

The hit takes the edge off, and I stare up at the stars through the window. The night is very clear so everything in the sky is in perfect view. A flash of Kristen's beautiful blond hair flutters through my mind and I fall asleep imagining my arms around her.

68. Conspiracy

It's noon. By now there's an outstanding arrest warrant attached to my name. I'm still at Jeremy's and I have no plans on leaving. I can't have any interaction with law enforcement. One check on my name will lead to arrest, and ultimately jail time I'm sure. I'll die before I dry out in another holding cell. There's no way. I still don't have any clue as to how I got through it a couple months ago. That was terrible, easily my worst nightmare come true. Thinking about it is enough to make me cringe – I'll do everything in my power to prevent it from happening again.

I find myself closing any blinds that are open on the windows in the house. I'm beginning to get a bit paranoid. The phone rang with an unrecognizable number and I pretty much ran in the other direction silently screaming. I keep thinking of weird convoluted ways that I can be traced here. What if they check out my brother for some reason and he gets followed here by an undercover cop? What if Jeremy says something stupid at work and that guy who knows Brad decides to give me up out of good measure? These thoughts are going through my head, and even though I realize they are ridiculous – they still freak me out. I wasn't prepared to be this paranoid about it all. I didn't expect that I'd even think about it this much. It's time to sit on the couch and chill out. There are no helicopters circling the house waiting for me to show myself. There are no secret FBI agents tapping the phone line listening to every word I say. There are no tracking devices installed on my brother's car that are going to lead all of the cops in the city here. The phone rings and I nearly fall off of the couch. I creep over to the edge of the coffee table and lift up the phone carefully to peek at the caller ID – it's my brother.

"Hey." I answer with a tone of exasperation.

"What's up with you? You sound all freaked out? I'm coming over." He says.

"Alright, I'll be here." And I hang up the phone.

I really need to calm down. I go to the small table in the corner of the room and slide out its tiny drawer. Rolling papers and a small baggie of weed is stashed away inside. I bring it all over to the coffee table and get to work rolling a gigantic joint. Maybe this will help with the anxiety; I need to stop thinking this crazy shit. I am hoping that my brother being here will help with it as well. Perhaps he'll have the ability to get my mind off of things long enough that I'll have a few minutes where I'm not looking over my shoulder toward the windows in the kitchen. For some reason I am convinced that the deck out back is going to be overridden by SWAT at any moment and tear gas canisters are going to be tossed in through the windows. I need to focus.

My brother shows up and immediately notices that I'm being nutty. He looks at me carefully before saying anything.

"Weren't you supposed to go to court this morning?" He asks me. There's really no point in lying to him, he'll just find out in the long run anyways, and besides, it's probably best if he knows that I can't afford to be found right now.

"I skipped out on it, and I need to stay under the radar for a little while, so keep me under your hat." I answer, trying to sound stern enough where he won't give me even more shit. He nods at me but I can tell that he really doesn't approve. His furrowed brow is only a small indication to the millions of thoughts he is currently processing behind it. In an instant he realizes all of the reasons that brought me to this decision. This is why I can trust him with shit, he'll get to the same place that I am and therefore have the ability to hold back the judgment. I hold out the joint to him and he takes it with pleasure pulling a lighter out from his pocket. He lights it carefully and takes what looks to be a much needed hit. Most likely due to the information I just dropped on him. He knows that it's really bad to skip out on court. He also knows that it's even worse to skip out on court when you got arrested the night before on a breaking and entering charge. He knows that I'll most likely end up in jail for this little stunt, but he also knows why that can't happen right now. He gets it all so completely, and he doesn't even have to tell me this – I can already tell.

He tells me that he's in between classes but isn't planning on going back to the college. This is the one day of the week where he avoids working completely, but makes up his time on the weekend so that he can still collect a full time salary. That gives us the entire afternoon to hang out, which will help me greatly. My paranoia has already calmed down since he walked in the door, and the joint was a very good idea. My brother tosses in a movie that we both like so that our background noise is at least somewhat intelligent and not filled with talk shows and bullshit news. I run to the kitchen and grab a couple of beers remembering that I stocked up the other day. It's a rarity for me to have the ability to offer anything to anyone else, so when I can it makes me happy inside. Sometimes I forget that I have anything though, because I am so unused to it. My brother seems surprised to see the beer appear before him, usually if he's drinking anything it's something that he brought over himself. He smiles at me and cracks it open.

We sit on the couch for the rest of the afternoon watching the movie from time to time and talking about mindless things. The time we spend is calm and not centered around my addiction or the arrest. It's the most comfortable I have felt since Brad first appeared on my doorstep. My brother takes it upon himself to order us up a pizza. I don't have a problem with the delivery guy coming to the house providing that I am out of view when he gets here, just in case he was to be interrogated in the future. I know that this is another crazy thought, but it's easy enough to duck into another room when he arrives rather than taking the chance. The knock at the door startles me a bit, but I just sneak into the hallway until I hear my brother shut the front door after paying for the food. He laughs at me as I make my way back out to the living room, I just ignore it and sit back down on the couch.

"I really don't think that Domino's is trying to track down your whereabouts." He says to me with slight amusement in his voice.

"Hey – I'm not taking chances with anything that is out of my control. No way." I reply shaking my head. He lets out another laugh and then opens up the pizza box on the coffee table. After getting high and throwing back a few beers the pizza actually sounds really good to me. I don't really remember the last time that I actually wanted to eat. Usually I just do it when I don't have a choice. When I can feel that my entire body is starting to have the shakes due to lack of energy and my stomach is stabbing me from within with hunger pains. That's when I finally break down and put something in my mouth that can be converted into energy by my rotten body. Actually having a desire or a craving for food however hasn't happened to me in a long time. It feels good to be able to satisfy my hunger like a normal person today. I have no idea why today is so special when it comes to my stomach, but I'm not going to ask any questions. Head down, I pick up a slice of pizza and touch it to my lips. The taste is exactly what I was expecting. It's not too hot anymore due to the travel, which is perfect because I can eat it without burning the inside of my mouth. There's nothing worse than scolding hot pizza sauce spurting out from underneath a blanket of cheese when you take that first bite. This doesn't happen though, instead I am overrun with satisfaction, which makes me happy, and surprises me all at the same time.

My brother is oblivious to this, and just continues eating pizza like he has never eaten before. He can really put some pizza away, I'll probably only have one more piece though, so it really makes no difference to me. He probably won't even leave any for Jeremy, which actually makes me laugh when I think about it, seeing as how Jeremy is usually the one supplying us with free pizza. The more I think about it the more I laugh inside.

An hour or so later my brother slowly comes to life on the couch and decides to stand up. He's going to go pick up his girlfriend, or so he announces, and he throws the pizza box away in the kitchen before leaving. I tell him that I'm going to stay right here for as long as I can and hide out. The door closes behind him and I see his headlights disappear down the long driveway. It's time for my first hit of the day. I walk down the hallway toward my room feeling my veins jump in the direction of the closet. A perfect ending to a perfect day, and I've made it without being captured.

69. Building

uccessfully hiding out is actually very easy. All you have to do to pull it off is never leave wherever you are staying. I have the craft down perfectly. I haven't left Jeremy's house for five straight days now, and I have no burning desire to do so in the near future. It's really too easy. Some people get cabin fever, but I can't even see that happening to me, at least not in this current state. I would rather be confined to this house for the rest of my life than risk getting locked up. I'm still convinced that it would kill me. I'm not physically or mentally able to handle going through withdrawal without medical assistance. It would rip me to shreds from the inside out. I'll do anything to prevent that from happening.

Jeremy seems to have no problem grabbing things on his way home from work if I desperately need something. That has only happened once though, and I actually had cash here to reimburse him for the bottle of vodka that I absolutely had to have. I'm sure that helped in his quick agreement to stop for me. Either way I haven't come up with a reason that could get me out of this house right now. I know what is going to get me out, but nobody else does yet. I'm planning on making my exit in about a week or so, until then everyone just needs to be patient with me. Everything is hinging on when I run out of dope and take that last hit.

My brother has been trying to make my time in seclusion as interesting as possible. He doesn't realize fully how much I don't mind staying here sheltered from the outside world. He thinks that I'm just not openly complaining about it, but the truth is that I actually enjoy it for the most part. I have no complaints at all at the moment, except for the obvious ones that never really go away. As far as my current situation goes, I'm perfectly content. I entertain his efforts though so as to not hurt his feelings. I feel bad though because he is trying so hard. He keeps making mix CD's and bringing over all these outdoors magazines that he knows I like. I have stacks and stacks of magazines that would literally take me months just to thumb through. After awhile I get tired of flipping the pages and give up on them for the day. He's really trying to make sure that I never have even the slightest shred of boredom to deal with.

I haven't spoken to anybody else in the last five days either. I think that Nikki has tried to call me, but the phone still freaks me out. It usually rings during the day when I'm the only one here, and I refuse to answer any number that I don't recognize. There have been a few repeat unrecognizable numbers that have shown up day after day, which leads me to believe that it might be Nikki. At the same time it freaks me out even more that perhaps it's someone related to the law in some way, and they have finally tracked me down. Perhaps they haven't fully tracked me down, but they have a lead at least that I might be hiding out here. It doesn't matter though, because I'm not ever going to answer it. If someone else happens to be here the next time it calls and they feel brave enough to pick it up – that's fine. I'll just find out then whatever fate awaits me on the other end of the call.

Fortunately though, the rest of the paranoia has pretty much disappeared. I don't watch over my shoulder anymore as I walk around the house. Unless they have invented x-ray vision and are looking down on us from the sky – nobody knows that I am in here. Cars drive by outside like normal and I am able to suppress the urge to run and hide underneath my bed. The phone is really the only thing left that still gives me the creeps. My stomach flops every single time that it rings, no matter what time of the day it is. The nervousness doesn't go away until the phone stops ringing or I know who is on the other end for sure. I don't think that I'm ever going to get over that damn phone. It's just too intrusive, too close. I hate it.

Another piece of good news is that I have still been able to keep my dope use under some kind of control. I have still not let myself spiral out of control with it, and I am locked into a pretty steady schedule. When I find myself wanting to slip from it and use before I should, I down some alcohol and stave off the craving. I figure that it's better to take a few drinks here and there than to give in to the addiction right away. I should at least try. This is the logic that I have been telling myself, and it seems to be working so far. I haven't even come close to slipping into the hole that I was in before my brother dragged me out of the apartment and brought me here a few weeks ago. Therefore I must be doing something right. As long as I can execute this next step in my plan – things are going to get better.

Evan has called the house a few times, but I have been staying away from him too. I don't need his influence right now, and he doesn't need mine. I need to stay away from every single person I know that has or currently uses heroin. I know that having someone else by my side just raises my chances of spiraling out of control again, and that's a move that I desperately cannot afford right now. I've cut it too close so many times as it is, I can't fuck this up. In a lot of ways I'm looking at this as my last shot. The need to focus has never been so important in my life, and is only going to get even more important as time pushes on. I'm going to have a lot of people counting on me soon, and it's going to take a lot in order to not disappoint. I can only hope that I have what it takes to get the job done. I have no credibility behind me, but I am at a different place right now, and I think that I have faith in myself for the very first time. I think that I actually believe it. I might be completely delusional right now, but I have felt this way for over two weeks now, and it doesn't seem to be going away.

Jeremy has found an apartment that he is planning on renting about five miles away from here. It's a small one bedroom apartment that he's going to use as a temporary home until he finds himself another house. Jeremy's simple lifestyle makes a house a perfect investment for him. He does everything so consistently and manages to build all kinds of equity in his property. This place is being purchased at an inflated rate as it is due to the extenuating circumstances. He'll be walking away from it with a pretty large chunk of change in his pocket. After he got over the initial shock of losing his house, this little fact started to sink into his head. I think he's actually looking forward to kissing the place goodbye at this point. He keeps talking about buying some land and just building a house, which I think is a great idea if he has the cash for it, which obviously he does. Aside from the occasional pizza he literally doesn't spend a dime. I bet he has a mountain of cash sitting in a bank somewhere, and now he's just going to add to it with the profit from this sale. He's going to be all set, which makes me happy. I just wish that somewhere along the way I had figured that shit out and done the same for myself, but I lack motivation. At least I know that.

In a very short period of time everything is going to change again. The people in my life will shift, and a new configuration will present itself. I'll begin a new cycle, and start new daily routines with new characters and places. Things seem to shift so quickly in my life, one minute I'm here, and the next I'm over there. With a blink of an eye I'm drying out in a holding cell, or walking around a rehab facility throwing tables and smashing coffee pots. From the truck to the apartment, to Jeremy's, to wherever. Every day brings on a new adventure that could change my course of life completely. The ride that I have been on has been rocky at times, and very high at others. As soon as it levels itself out and slows down for just a few minutes – I'll take a deep breath and step off of it forever.

70. Finality

The last few days have been sad, and a little weird. Jeremy had a mental breakdown in the kitchen the other day and started throwing things in a fit of rage. He has periods here and there when he loses it completely. He can't accept that his house is about to be demolished in just a couple more days. I thought that he was going to bring the entire kitchen down himself when he threw his little tantrum, but it's still standing. He has put his fist through a few of the walls just to have some fun, it's all going to be run over by heavy machinery soon anyways, so it doesn't make a difference. I took a sledgehammer to the inside wall of my room. I must admit, it felt really good to destroy something.

I have been using up my supply right on schedule, slowly depleting the heaping amount with each day that passes. I have only had a few bad days where I felt the onslaught of depression, but I was able to keep it together for the most part and work through it. I have a pretty good supply of alcohol built up still, which still continues to help with the constant cravings. All in all everything has lined up so well, I just have to take the last leap. From this point on, everything is completely up to me.

My hide out is about to be whisked away from underneath me. I've decided to not return to the apartment. Nikki and I are going to be very bad news for each other at this time. I'm going to avoid that whole situation completely, which should be easy because I already have another plan in mind. It's the same plan that I have had ever since I went and made my last big score. It's the scariest plan that I have ever constructed on my own, but I think I'm finally ready.

I allowed Evan to come down last night and hang out with Jeremy and my brother. It was a little gathering to bid the place goodbye once and for all. Pizza was had, three of them to be exact, and many empty beer bottles later – we were all passed out in the living room. Evan got up this morning bright and early because he had to be to work by 9:00am in order to cook a banquet lunch of some sort. My brother just left about an hour ago after missing his first class of the day. He mumbled something about just going straight to work and blowing off the entire day of classes. I don't think that he really needs to show up for half of his classes anyways, he seems to be able to pass them without much work on his part at all. Jeremy got up right at the crack of dawn as usual and went straight to work – as usual. I think it was about 5:30am when I heard the van outside start up. He always puts his responsibilities first.

I am now sitting here all alone on the couch staring off into space trying to collect my thoughts. Trying to collect my strength. My stomach is knotted in anticipation and my head is spinning like a top. I have set forth some goals for myself, and I need to follow through with them – just this one time I have to actually put some effort it and give it my all. I owe it to myself. I owe it to many others as well.

I want to see Kristen soon. I want to let her know that I'm not upset for what she did the next morning after I overdosed at her house. I want her to know that I'm glad she did what she did, and that I don't hold anything against her. She did not betray my trust in any way, and I still love her dearly, as I always will. I need to see her, but now is not the right time. Seeing her now would be unfair to her and unfair to me as well. I have to do this first. I have to execute my plan first.

I need to see my mother soon as well. I have to let her know that I'm ok, and that I can take care of myself. That I'm not just going to waste away on the side of the road like some nasty stinking junkie. I'm not going to rob people and hurt anyone anymore than I already have. I can be trusted. I can be compassionate and nice. I can be an upstanding human being that makes correct decisions. I can handle responsibility. I can actually exist in a manner that doesn't hurt others. These are all of the things that I need to prove.

I need to stop running away from the things that cause me pain. I need to actually deal with some of it before jumping on the needle. Heroin is not the answer to life's problems. I just need to find a way to believe that. I need to pull myself up off of the floor and kick my own ass around the entire house. I need to throw myself through the walls and use my body as a wrecking ball until I realize that I just can't do this shit anymore. I can't do it to myself and I can't do it to all of the people around me. I can't.

I spring to my feet instantly. Before I know it I am running down the hallway and into my room. The closet is glowing and pulsating with soft light. I fall at the pile of clothes and start throwing them in all directions until I uncover the little wooden box. I pick it up gently and cradle it in my arms. I finally have the nerve built up inside of me; I have to do this now before it's too late. Before the feeling fades and goes away. Before another part of me makes the wrong decision – again.

I find my way back on the couch in the living room in what seems like an instant. As if I blinked my eyes and appeared here out of thin air. The house has started to look a bit strange because most of the furniture has already been moved to Jeremy's new apartment. This makes the open spaces seem very large and at times overwhelming. Perhaps that only affects me – it wouldn't surprise me if that was the case.

I set the wooden box down on the coffee table and push everything else there on the floor. Remotes, bottles, pizza boxes, papers, plates, napkins, an ashtray, even a half full 40 – all on the floor. I need this time to concentrate. I need myself and this box to be the only two things in this room that matter. I need to say goodbye. I have a piece of paper folded up in my pocket that I have been carrying around with me for two weeks waiting for just the right time. Waiting for my supply to be low enough. I pull it out and dial the number that is written on it as quickly as I can - cringing as I wait for someone to answer on the other end. Two minutes later I hang up the phone and set it down next to me on the couch. I stare at the wooden box for another ten minutes or so before I slide it toward me slowly and open it up. One metal cap, one brand new needle, one small little bit of heroin. It's all I have left, and it's all I need.

I cook it up and load the syringe. I pick up the phone again and dial my brother.

"Hey – I reserved a bed at rehab, come get me before I change my mind." I hang up the phone before he can even answer. One last long stare into the eyes of my poisonous lover. One last taste of her sweet nectar. All of the pain in the world disappears, and a great sadness washes over me, as I say goodbye to her once and for all.

71. Transition

'm almost two months clean, and life has never been so hard. I found employment in the convenience store portion of a chain gas station. It's a ten minute walk from the room I am renting down the street for $75 a week. I'm paying for it on my own with the money that I make at the little store. I haven't missed a day of work since I started about a month ago. I haven't even been late for that matter.

Nikki is living on her own back at the apartment and has successfully stayed away from heroin. She has however revisited her old friend Cocaine a few times, and still struggles with the bulimia. She only throws up after certain meals now – I'm sure that she'll end up back in the hospital in due time. Unfortunately right now there really isn't anything that I can do for her. Last time I visited her we got into a pretty heated argument. I suspect that it will be awhile before we see each other again. It's best for both of us if we keep some distance for right now. The cleaner we are the harder it is for us to deal with each other it seems. It's sad really, but I can't really figure out a solution that works, so for the time being – I'm on my own, and so is she.

Rehab wasn't too bad to deal with, but I went in with a slightly better attitude than ever before. I still found the groups, and the counselors, and the psychobabble completely useless and extremely unhelpful, but the meds to help with the withdrawal is what got me there. I knew that I wasn't going to be able to pull it off on my own. I had already made up my mind before going in that I wanted to finally kick it and be clean. I needed the time to detox, and I needed to do it correctly with medical aid. Getting locked up or running out of shit would have killed me physically. I had to go into this with some help, and knew what I needed this time in order to facilitate a chance of success. I never thought for one second that I would willingly call the rehab facility and schedule myself a bed. I never thought that I would take that step unless it was forced upon me against my will. I suppose that makes all the difference in the world – having the strength and ability to make that decision on my own. I suppose that was a sign that told me I was actually ready to do this, and to do it right. I kept my head down while I was in there, fulfilling the things that were required of me, but doing nothing extra. I didn't make friends, and I wasn't an exceptional patient. I didn't cause trouble or even bother talking most of the time. I blocked it all out and stayed on course with what I knew was right in my head. I don't need to be brainwashed into thinking like a completely different person. I don't need to turn into the biggest spokesperson against heroin, or any other substance for that matter. I just needed to curve my addiction and find a way to avoid the substances that control me. That's all. No magical wand is going to take away my mental dependencies to heroin. No counselor who has been clean for fifteen years yelling at me about all of his fucked up experiences is going to help me kick my habit. Perhaps it works for other people – and that's great, but for me I have to be the one who changes my mind. I'm the only one who can keep me on the right track and away from these horrible things that turn my life to shit. It's been beyond hard. Harder than words can even describe. Almost every thought that I have is consumed with that of using again. The needles, the packets, the metal caps, the sounds of it cooking up, the smell of the flame from the lighter after it has lit steadily for thirty seconds. Everything surrounding my addiction hits me square in the face almost every single minute of every single day. I deal with it as it comes and try to get my mind off of it as soon as it shows up. It's a struggle every time though, and I fear that it will continue to be. I'm never going to feel the same as I did before I started using. I think that I have accepted that, at least I have so far. If I can just keep going strong, I'll be all set.

I no longer have to hide from the law anymore; as soon as I got cleaned up in rehab I went and turned myself in. There's something that I never thought I'd say or do, but I did. I knew that I was going to need to get a job in order to support myself, and there was no way of doing that without clearing up that outstanding arrest warrant first. Surprisingly they went somewhat easy on me. I got fifteen days in jail which was cut down from a thirty day sentence originally. Apparently they viewed my act of turning myself in as noble, and decided to give me a break. I'll take it. The fifteen days in jail was boring, but really not that bad to deal with at all. Having already gone through drying out, and in a much more humane manner, there was really nothing to worry about while being locked up, except for actually being locked up. It takes a few days to get used to it, but after that it's a piece of cake. I wouldn't want to serve twenty years or anything like that, but fifteen days wasn't all that bad. I got slapped with five years probation due to my record of possession charges and a few larceny charges. That's fine with me too; probation doesn't bother me at all.

After I got all of that taken care of I got myself a room in a giant building full of rooms near downtown. My mother hooked me up with a couple of week's worth of rent to get me going, and I set out on day one looking for a job within walking distance. I landed at the gas station which is on the corner of my street and another heavily traveled road that crosses it. They hired me the next day after I filled out the application and left it with the manager. My duties basically consist of running one of the registers up front and cleaning up around the store near the end of my shift every night. The store is open until midnight and I usually work the last shift. That gives me the entire day to do whatever I want, and since I'm not a morning person I get to sleep as late as I like. For right now, this configuration has been the most successful for me out of all the others that I have tried so desperately to work in the past. I don't mind working as much as I used to. I don't mind my shitty little room that I live in. I don't mind all of the drunken assholes that also live there. I find that nothing really bothers me all that much anymore. I just keep to myself and stay out of trouble. At some point I can hopefully turn my life around so that it is actually productive enough where I can build a future for myself. Right now though I am just focusing on staying clean. That's my second job, and it gets top priority. If I fuck that up, then everything else is going to crumble to the ground, and quickly. I already know this from past experiences; I could be considered an expert on it really so basically I have no excuses anymore.

     I have been trying to get outside more as well, seeing as how the tundra like weather is starting to subside, and there really isn't anything to do in my little tiny room. There are a few parks near my street that have some small trails which weave in and out of the woods that border them. I walk them from time to time enjoying the nature that surrounds me. It's nothing like what I am used to, but until I have steady transportation I am just going to have to use my resources as best I can. The dirty homeless people that frequent my street at night tend to stay away from me when I'm walking home from work. When they don't get out of my way I shoot them dirty looks to let them know what they'd be getting into if they started shit. The degenerates around here are pussies for the most part, nothing compared to the scum that walk around the magical city where I used to score. Those guys will fuck you up and spit you out, as I have already experienced firsthand. These idiots around here are just looking for a handout so they can get more booze. I don't have a very good tolerance for drunks. There are so many other wonderful drugs out there to get addicted to; I never really understood the alcohol thing. I loved using it to curve my cravings, but I couldn't imagine being hooked on it the way some of these people are. I guess everybody has their own thing though.

Standing Room Only

There is one window above the mattress that I have in my tiny little room. The floor is pretty grimy, but I did my best cleaning it with a borrowed rug cleaner before I moved in. It's still pretty stained with unidentifiable things, but for the most part I just try to stay away from it. It's not really a place that you'd like to go barefoot in. My mattress is actually a futon mattress that a friend of mine gave me when I got out of rehab. He was replacing it with another futon, and this one is in beautiful condition – I love it. It's my favorite possession at the moment. I can see the sun slowly starting to set from behind me as it shines in through the window above my head. I am sitting on the edge of the mattress peacefully staring at the opposite wall. Tenants in these places come and go almost every day. The walls in every room tell a story. For the most part none of these stories can be deciphered, but they are there nonetheless. My walls are covered with scribblings from markers, pens, pencils, spray paint, crayon, charcoal – you name it. Every inch of paint has been replaced with someone's masterpiece. Someone's piece of artwork that will only be seen by each subsequent occupant. I can't help but think of how wasteful this is. How the talent that lives behind these pieces will never be discovered or put out into the real world. They will never be utilized the way that they should be, they will never be seen by those who should see them. It makes me wish that I could see everyone else's room just to lay eyes on the artwork that lives inside of each one. Just to give each drawing a life, even if it's in my own head. Just to give all of the talent floating around in this building justice and permanency. It makes me think of my friend that died just a few months ago.

I throw on my hoodie and gather up my things that I will need for my shift at work. Wallet, smokes, lighter, keys – that's it. Slipping into my shoes I take one last scan around the small room in case I'm forgetting something that I just can't live without during the next six hours. I'm pretty confident that I have everything – I always have that feeling like I am forgetting something, but I attribute it to the lack of my precious wooden box. I pull my hood up over my head and turn the knob to my door locking it behind me – it's time to go to work.

72. Maintain

Working hasn't been nearly as bad as it used to be. Wanting to be on the outside to use so badly – played a significant role in my defiance. I still don't like the concept very much, but it doesn't bother me quite as much. My shifts go by pretty quickly for the most part, and my brother stops in every couple of days to hang out with me for a bit outside. That's usually when I take one of my smoke breaks for the night. A strange crowd frequents this gas station at night. Since it's on the corner of two somewhat busy streets it sees a lot of faces. The cops have been here for a few flare ups in the parking lot between patrons, but other than that there doesn't really seem to be much trouble.

After work I usually just walk back to my room and sleep eventually. Sometimes I sit on the edge of my bed and flip through a rock climbing magazine, I'm still nowhere near close to getting through the stacks that my brother used to bring for me when I was staying at Jeremy's. I've been glad that I have them though, because there really isn't anything to do in my room. I got my hands on a cheap boom box that I have plugged into one of the two outlets that I posses. This helps me get to sleep at night – I usually play something nice and quiet while I fall asleep. It helps me to get my mind off of all the other sudden noises that creep up out of nowhere through the night. There are some strange characters that live here. I want to find another place to move to soon, but for now it's perfect. I keep to myself and don't bother anybody, which seems to be key.

Everyone is starting to get used to my sobriety. They finally all actually believe that I am clean. I suppose it was never hard to identify that I wasn't in the past at certain times. The difference between my life then and now is exponential. This makes me feel good, and is honestly the only thing that continues to give me the strength I need to stay clean. They're my motivation. I'm not sure if any of them know this, but without their support it would be an impossible task. It practically is anyways – I'm not sure how I will ever stop missing that horrible substance. Every corner presents a test, and so far I have been able to pass with flying colors.

I still haven't hooked up with Kristen since I got clean. I'm ashamed with myself and can't seem to get past it. My mother has kept in contact with her apparently and keeps her updated on my condition, but I haven't actually spoken to her myself. I need to get over it and see her, I owe her that much at least, not to mention I miss her to death. I keep over thinking things though and turn into too much of a perfectionist when it comes to her. I want to make sure that everything is all lined up and in perfect order before I see her. I can't risk failing right before her eyes all over again.

That's pretty much my biggest worry these days – making amends with certain people. Other than that my life has been pretty dull actually. I'm living the lifestyle that I always protested in the pas. At the moment it's the only thing that will work for me so I don't really have a choice. I'm realizing now that in order to have been able to live the life that I wanted was to put some real effort into things in the beginning. I didn't do this. I didn't know then that it would ultimately be the deciding factor for my future.

I feel like another sheep that's out there walking around – accomplishing menial tasks and barely getting by. My pockets are always void of cash even though I live in an eight foot by ten foot box. I don't spend money on anything except for smokes and the occasional descent meal. For the most part I eat very affordable items like boxed pasta. I rarely splurge, and there really isn't anything that I want. The only thing that I want is the ability to get ahead in life and live somewhere halfway descent. I would like to have my own apartment someday and a job that actually pays a respectable salary. That's pretty much all I am looking for, but I can't seem to figure out how to get there.

My room is equipped with two closets, one smaller than the main one. The large one has a few of my shirts hanging in it and then my backpack and camping gear stored on the floor. The smaller one has nothing except for some books on the floor in two neat stacks. Aside from my futon mattress, and a giant black chest that I had in my room at my mother's house, there's nothing else to be seen. The chest basically gets used as my table so I keep it close to the bed. Glasses go there, and so do my keys, which I only have a few hanging on a metal ring. Smokes, lighter, and ashtray can also be found there, next to a small lamp that I found in the corner of the small closet when I moved in. It's simple, and perfect. If only I had just a few more rooms to call my own.

The kitchen is communal and each floor has one. It's considered bad etiquette to stray from your kitchen and use another floor's. This isn't like a large house that has been subdivided. It's literally a building full of rooms and hallways that are identical from one floor to another. Bathroom and kitchen is shared by everyone else on your floor. I do my best to not think about the sanitary issues this must raise. I also do my best to bum showers at other people's houses whenever I can. I have gotten away with a few at Evan's house recently and a few over at Nikki's of course. The shower here isn't really that bad, but the thought of some of the people who use it freaks me out. Although some of the people look like they have never showered in their lives, so perhaps only the clean ones are using the shower. Either way it still freaks me out. I touch nothing when I am in there, and I go as fast as humanly possible – while dying inside myself.

Some nights are extremely hard to get to sleep. Tonight is one of those nights. I can hear faint music and muffled televisions buzzing in every direction. The person upstairs just got up and paced around their room for about ten minutes straight. The guy below me has been throwing up for the last forty-five minutes. I hope that he has a bucket or something that he's doing it in at least. These aren't the things that are preventing me to sleep though. In fact, they don't bother me at all, they're simply observations that I am forced to make due to a sudden blast of insomnia. The reason I can't get to sleep is because I can't stop thinking about getting high. I relive the feeling over and over again, and yearn to let it take me away. I roll around on the mattress and fight back the urge to destroy the giant black chest to my left. My muscles spasm uncontrollably waiting for me to make a move, but I can't. I'm trapped inside my own insanity. I'm stapled to the floor waiting for the craving to pass. I want to feel it more than anything else in the world.

As soon as it starts to feel safe I slowly move my arms and legs. I have an enormous bottle of vodka stashed in my backpack on the closet floor a few feet away. I stretch out toward it and drag the bag over to the bed, sweat pouring off of my forehead. I get myself so worked up just by thinking about the shit. I pull out the bottle and struggle with the cap for what seems like hours before downing as much as I can handle in one swig. I don't drink out of the blue – I drink when it gets really bad. The truth is I don't really like alcohol enough to turn it into an addiction. It certainly works better than anything else though when it comes to this, therefore it has its place. I don't believe that drinking occasionally will turn me into a heroin addict again like most people do, so I allow myself to use it whenever I see fit. I get two more big swigs in me before I start to calm down enough to move freely. I'm hoping that it just makes me tired enough so that I can get more than three hours of sleep tonight. The last few nights have been rougher than usual and I have been waking up on the hour. I only hit the bottle twice last night and was hoping that tonight would be a little bit better. So far that doesn't seem to be the case.

The guy downstairs has finally quieted down with all of the puking noises – my brother would have been dying during that whole spiel. I don't think that I have heard the person upstairs for about an hour or so either – they must have finally chilled out and decided to go to bed. I have no idea what time it is, but I got here around 12:30am and it feels like I've been laying here for days. I know that I haven't though; it's probably only about 2:00am. I cap the bottle and roll back over on my other side. It's a little bit colder than usual tonight so I make sure that my sleeping bag is completely zipped up. This is what I use to sleep in on top of the futon mattress. It's my camping sleeping bag that was still at my mother's house – I love how warm it keeps you.

I fill my head with positive thoughts. Kristen getting ready for work in the morning. The cool blast of fresh air that you feel the first time you step foot out of your house. A blazing hot coffee and that perfect first smoke of the day. Sleep comes to me quickly, and holds me down soundly for the entire night.

73. Dining

My brother is coming over today to hang out and eventually give me a ride to work. It's one of those unusual days where he managed to evade school and work at the same time. He found a loophole somewhere and took it – that's what he does. I certainly have no complaints as I was planning on just sitting around my room all day. It's freezing outside so there was really no point in going out and trying to find a nice trail to walk. At least now I'll have some company. He's been here already a few times in the last month, but never really with anytime to stay. His schedule has been nuts with the new semester that just started. Juggling classes in order to maintain a forty hour work week is a difficult task to pull off – but he does it. I never could. I never cared enough to even bother. The thought of it alone discouraged me, and so I just never tried. I still have no desire to be that assertive when it comes to schooling and work. I have a feeling that he is actually doing all of this now to get it out of the way. Precisely what I wish I was smart enough to do. Oh well.

I meet him outside so that we can walk up to my room together; it's weird getting used to finding it. Once inside I shut the door and take a seat back down on the futon. We both decide, over a smoke, that it's time to make some food. We are going to brave the communal kitchen down the hall. I grab the small pot that I have in the corner of the closet and a couple packages of Ramen noodles – the cornerstone of any nutritious meal. All we need to whip this tasty meal up is some water from the beat up sink in the kitchen. I grab the wooden spoon that I have stashed in my room, and we make our way down the hallway together.

The kitchen has really been abused by the people here. The stove is electric and therefore equipped with four coil-type burners. Every single one of them is physically broken, which makes the coil itself slanted and halfway falling inward toward the stove. They all still work oddly enough, but just cause your pot or pan to be tilted the entire time that you use the burner. I can only imagine what the oven portion must look like, and have never had the courage to open it. I will stick to my Ramen noodles, fast, easy, and with no chance of touching anything except for the pan that I brought in with me. My brother and I hover over by the stove together and wait for the water to boil.

The kitchen itself is extremely small. It is about the size of what you would picture a laundry room to be – a narrow rectangle with a fridge on one side and a stove on the other. A nasty sink is in between the two, mounted on the wall, and reminds you more of a bathroom sink than one you would find in a kitchen. While we are standing there random people come in and put things in the fridge, others come and retrieve things, mostly drinks of some sort – never alcohol. That shit gets hidden away in people's rooms, they wouldn't risk it getting stolen – and it would get stolen. I'm sure that half of the bottles of Mountain Dew in there end up getting stolen – alcohol wouldn't stand a chance.

There is a small round wooden table next to the stove that has a couple of magazines strewn about on it. They seem quite tattered and don't look like anything a clean person would want to touch. My brother and I continue to stand on opposite sides of the stove staring at the never boiling water. Neither of us are speaking, and we haven't since we got in here. A strange atmosphere is surrounding just the two of us. We are both on guard for anything and constantly aware of whomever is around. We are attentive to every little detail and every little change in the room, or even outside in the hallway for that matter. I can tell that we are both thinking the same thoughts. We are both making the same assessments in our heads at the same exact time. It's an odd feeling to describe. We have had a lot of moments together, but nothing like this before. It's weird how certain bonds just get stronger throughout time.

The water finally starts to boil and I dump in two of the packages of noodles. This part doesn't usually take all that long – soon enough we will be out of here and back in the room. Another person comes slinking in behind my brother babbling something about the fire alarm. We look at each other trying not to laugh until the guy finally stumbles back out into the hallway. It's always so hard to not laugh right in people's faces when it's the two of us together. The noodles are about done anyways. I reach over and shut off the burner while bringing the pot over to the sink to drain all of the excess water out. My brother stands by the doorway waiting for me – still silent.

All done with the draining – we head back to the room. Door shut and locked, all is well once again. The outside craziness is confined to their specific areas and completely out of view. I have a small arsenal of utensils, and surprisingly two ceramic bowls. I split up the noodles and put the pan down by the door so as to remember to wash it when we are done. My brother digs right into his portion as I mess around with the boom box for a minute. The traffic outside seems heavy – it must be getting close to five. The noodles seem to disappear from both of our bowls rather quickly – it's time to fill the room with smoke. My brother surprises me and pulls out a joint just like old times. I haven't smoked in a couple of weeks so this will be a fun treat. My brother lights it up and gets us going, the smell fills the room instantly and I am immediately thrown into a relaxed state of mind. I feel like freezing this moment – just like all of the others that I have wanted to freeze in the past. This is one of those times.

My brother motions toward the door – reminding me that it's almost time for me to go to work – he's eager to take a ride and get out of here for a little while – I don't blame him. I pile up the dishes in the corner and start putting on some layers.

Fortunately I'll only be walking one way from the store tonight, and there's a possibility that my brother will show up to drive me home too, he's done it a bunch of times in the past.

We make our way out to his car passing a few questionable looking people in the hallway as we walk to the stairwell. My brother has a knack for letting people know not to fuck with him. He stared them down as we walked past and I saw all three of them turn their heads in unison. He's good to have around, I could have used him when I was homeless, but that never would have worked out. He would have kicked my ass if he knew the shit that was going on out there. Those days are in the past now though – they're all behind me.

My brother starts up the car which he parked right in front of the building on the busy street. He punches it and squeals the tires a bit just to be an asshole as we pull away from the group of people that have congregated around the entrance to the building. The cops love checking this building throughout the day. There always seems to be something shady going on. It must be like a little playground for thcm, hoodlums standing on every corner of its brick construction. I stay out of the eyes of the law as much as possible. Fucking cops have done enough to make my life shit; I don't ever want anything to do with them ever. I continue to have no use for them in my life; even if I was being shot I wouldn't call those cocksuckers. Fuck it I'd rather take matters into my own hands. I certainly wouldn't want someone that I can't even trust trying to help me. My brother scoffs as we drive by a cruiser camped out on the busy street – his radar detector playing a symphony on the dashboard. I guess it runs in the family.

After a short drive around the city my brother pulls up to the store to drop me off. I run inside and return with a pack of smokes for him – just to hook him up for the ride and everything; he thanks me and heads off in the other direction.

Dining

The noodles are starting to give me heartburn, lucky for me – I work at a convenience store.

74. Empty

Each day is one more step in the right direction. I have to keep telling myself this in order to actually do it. Lately getting up out of bed is a chore in itself, because I am bored, and have nothing to really look forward to. I get up and do the same things every day, and I don't really have any idea why. I know that there are certain "normal" tasks which I must perform like everyone else in order to stay clean and keep myself on the right track. It just doesn't make anything easier. In fact it makes everything harder. I feel like that rat stuck in the metal wheel running at lightning speed, but never actually getting anywhere. My life has basically stopped – but I'm alive.

I spent the holidays in rehab, which is somewhat ironic because I spent last New Year's in rehab as well – so that makes two in a row. I even knew what to expect when New Year's rolled around. This time I didn't win anything in the scavenger hunt, but that's because I didn't bother to participate. It was weird being there for Christmas though. I imagined my tiny little family all congregating at my grandparent's house in the morning. My brother sitting on the couch drinking a coffee and waiting for gifts to be passed his way. My grandfather getting the fireplace ready so as to burn all of the wrapping paper that ends up flying around the room. All of the systems in place – I sat in my room in rehab thinking about heroin. Thinking about the life that I was never going to be able to have with Nikki. Thinking about how everything surrounding my addiction brings my life to a complete halt, but at the same time keeps it going. When it comes to heroin – I just can't seem to win. It is always going to be a thorn in my side, whether I am using or not, I just have to find a way to live with that knowledge.

I still have the little wooden box packed away in my backpack – it's empty now though. It's one of those things that I just can't seem to get rid of. The counselors at rehab would be really against me keeping it – but fuck them. I don't see how the idea of the wooden box can hurt me any less than actually having it. Some of the rules that these people come up with are whacky and have no basis in reality. I will never understand how we are so quick to develop systems based on nothing. If only I had the power to tear it all down. Then things could be rebuilt from the ground up, and possibly with some common sense and logic behind them this time. All of these great ideas, and I work at a gas station.

Nikki wants me to swing by her place later if I have time. I haven't decided if I am going to or not. Evan has also been showing himself more often, and giving me the option of staying at his place whenever I want. The only downside is that I have to find a way back here if I have to work the next day, but he always insists that he'll return me. I just haven't really felt all that social lately. I don't feel like being studied when I hang out, it seems that everyone has their eyes on me looking for signs of heroin use. That shit doesn't fly well with me. I do everything that I can to understand where they are coming from, but at the same time it gets a little discouraging, and exhausting to deal with. It makes me just want to scream at the top of my lungs "I'm not fucking using again!!!" Instead I just sit there and wait for it to pass. One of these days I'm going to go crazy and piss somebody off, I know it. I don't care though – at least I'm staying clean.

If I end up going to Nikki's place later we are just going to get in a fight – it's almost inevitable at this point. Last time we got into it because I asked her about her sudden reintroduction to coke. She's in complete denial about it and doesn't think that it's going to affect anything – this is what addicts do. I know this, because I use to do it all the time. I would get out of rehab and then find a way to rationalize my heroin use so that I didn't feel like I was ruining anything. I would tell myself that this time was going to be different. This time I was going to manage it better and do certain things differently. This time I was going to prevent it from throwing me into the fire pit. This time I was going to win, and this time I was going to be able to hold on to that wonderful feeling for as long as I want. I was always wrong. There is no "this time". You either use or you don't, and that's the end of it.

Her coke use is obviously contributing to her bulimia issues as well. Granted she has been able to somewhat control her obsessive vomiting, but she still engages in the act way too much. The doctors at the hospital told her that if she didn't straighten out her eating disorder she would eventually ruin every single organ in her body. Things were bad enough when she was in there – I can't believe that she would continue to behave in that manner. She knows that the bulimia is physically more dangerous to her right now than the drug use – but she still does it. Her stint as "most perfect person on the planet" has subsided finally, but she denies that her drug use right now is having any sort of negative effect on her life. She's pretty much gone right back to being the same Nikki, and it's so incredibly hard for me to stay away from her.

Seeing coke in her place doesn't bother me. The high from coke in comparison to heroin is so entirely different that I can't even compare the two. Coke has had its time and place here and there in my life, but that's it. Otherwise I can take it or leave it, and most of the time I chose to leave it. I'm glad that she's not back on heroin though – I wouldn't be able to handle that. If I walked into her place and she was cooking up a shot I would literally have to run in the opposite direction in order to avoid using. The sight of it would make my eyes bulge out of my skull and my feet hover over to wherever it was. I would be completely drawn to it, and unable to contain myself. I find myself staring off into space sometimes envisioning the process over and over again in my head. It's haunting to say the least, and requires endless concentration to get through. At least I don't have that to deal with though, I'm not sure if I'll ever even see that shit in person again. Let's hope not.

I have a payphone downstairs right outside the front door to the building, which surprisingly is usually easy to get on. You would think that with all of the scumbags living here, and the street itself being as busy as it is, that someone would always be using it, but no. I can pretty much get to it whenever I want with no problem at all. I have the ability to send my brother a numeric message on his pager without even using any money on the phone, which is very useful. I find myself struggling to keep change around; I never really have any loose coins on my person. I decide to give Evan a ring and see if he wants to hang out tonight when I get out of work. I figure I'll take him up on his incessant offers and get out of the city for a little while. I don't have to work tomorrow so there's no worry when it comes to a ride, and I'm sure he'll need to come down here for something anyways. It will be fun, and I haven't been to his place in a very long time it seems. He still lives with his parents, but they have pretty much given him the entire basement of the house to live in. It's the same footprint as the house itself and quite large – a really cool place actually. Evan agrees to pick me up at midnight in an instant – he must really want some company.

I run back up into my room as I have a few hours to kill before I need to go in for my shift. I am definitely not going over to Nikki's place later, something about it just seems wrong today, so I'll deal with her complaints tomorrow. I need to get away for the evening and chill out with a friend. I need some human interaction in another setting to break me free from this constant monotony. I need to feel a sense of belonging even if it's coming from the basement at Evan's house. I need a reminder as to why I am putting myself through a world of mental pain with every tick of the clock. I need a dose of justification that encourages me to keep going forward with this plan – and that it will pay off someday in the future. I need to feel something closer to love.

75. Reminiscing

Hanging out at Evan's house is going to be really good for me. It's exactly what I need at this time. Walking into the basement again felt so wonderful. The familiar incense smell hits me in the face as soon as I open the door at the top of the stairs. That smell brings me right back to some of my fondest memories. Evan and his brother used to be key members of a local band. They would jam in the far corner of this very basement almost every night. We would all be here hanging out and listening to their sessions. It was one of the best times of my life. Never a conflict and plenty of ridiculous laughter. It was a place where you could just be yourself and feel safe while doing so. Your voice could be heard and people would actually listen. A sanctuary that we created collectively and maintained at the highest level. Unfortunately – things change.

Not much about the basement itself has changed in all these years. It has just shrunken in on itself a little bit. Evan has fully furnished one half of it essentially turning it into a cross between a studio and loft apartment. The opposite wall has turned into a storage area of sorts, but a very neat storage area. Not much space has been taken up and the boxes that do exist are carefully stacked in planned order. The old days are gone and that half of the basement doesn't really get much use anymore. At least I have the memories.

Another very cool thing about the basement is that it comes fully equipped with a bathroom. Evan's parents had a bathroom installed a long time ago when they were kids because they anticipated a lot of future basement use. His parents are really cool people and always entertained our craziness. Their philosophy was as long as it wasn't hurting anybody – why not? I always really liked their approach.

Glimpses of my life from the pre-dope days give me hope. Hope of attaining happiness without the aid of a substance. I was able to do it in the past, which leads me to believe that I have a chance of getting back there. These reminders are good, and help with my overall lack of motivation to stay clean. My family members are the only reasons why I have gotten this far – I need something else. I'll hold onto these old memories for as long as I can as proof that my goal is reachable. It's just a matter of how much work and effort I am able to put into it. That's the key.

As I get closer to the bottom of the wooden stairs I can see the old table, we used to sit around all night long, leaning up against the wall of the basement. A million different nights flash through my head. The table still in the same place with only the faces sitting around it changing in configuration with each night that passes. Sometimes there were cards flying around the table as we played poker dressed up as characters that we had created. I remember my outfit being "redneck Joe", which came to life when I put on the red button down flannel and John Deer foam hat. Everyone added their own uniqueness to the game – it was a really cool time.

I point to the table as we walk by and Evan lets out a small chuckle remembering some of the more eventful nights. There were always a few that stuck out and got talked about over and over again and from each person's perspective. Trading stories like that back in forth with the players involved for some reason makes everyone feel really good. I love the groups of people that I used to spend all of my free time with. We created small dysfunctional families and treated each as such. We all had our roles and stuck to them as best we could, slipping at times, only to be caught by the next person in line. These are the relationships that people only dream about having. These are the bonds that some never even get the chance to experience. I feel honored to have at least lived it, and tasted it. I should have tried to keep the glue together, but I failed and know better now. If the situation ever arises again – I'll know what to do. Evan plops down on his bed and flips on the stereo lighting a smoke.

I brought over my gigantic sleeping bag which makes me feel like I never left my home in the first place. I'm lucky that I have gotten so accustomed to sleeping in it – It makes me very mobile – at least in an overnight situation. I open it up and spread it out on the floor a few feet away from Evan's bed. The night is young still – only about 12:40am – Evan pulls out his three foot plastic bong from around the side of his bed. He tosses me a baggie of weed since I'm already on the floor and I pack the bowl. I wasn't expecting this little treat. I pull out a lighter and Evan get's it burning. The smell is nice and adds to the atmosphere of the basement. I anticipate sleeping like a baby tonight.

Evan turns the music up a little bit louder – loud enough so that we don't disturb his parents too much – they actually work every day like normal people. The high from the weed is pure and perfect – easing me into a very relaxed state. My head drifts along with the music and Evan just sits there smiling at a thought in his head. Evan still has all of the same smatterings hanging on the walls which we all contributed to throughout the years. Strange drawings and hand written notes are hanging all over the place – as they always have. They are even all in the same spots as they used to be. Everything seems completely untouched like the bulletin board behind the counter of an old local diner. Evan's room was a time capsule of a life that I used to live. All of the elements were right there staring me in the face around every corner of the basement that I rediscovered. All of these images and memories were thrown on the back burner in the wake of using heroin. These wonderful experiences which helped mold me into the person I have become were overrun by thoughts of chasing a feeling. Chasing a feeling all the way down the longest tunnel in existence. There have been times where nothing in the world would have been able to stop me from using. I would have followed a needle right out in front of a speeding bus if that's what it took to have it. It pains me to think that heroin has made me forget about so many good things that I once had in life. I threw it at all away many times just to get my hands on that drug. Just to initiate that feeling one more time, and make the pain that bleeds through constantly – go away in an instant. Having that power and ability in my hands was impossible to not abuse.

There is speculation that the two of us are going to go for hike tomorrow. I brought my remaining gear with me which I was able to salvage from my mother's house a few weeks ago when I got out of jail. Evan's house is located about four miles away from my mother's so we are right in the middle of the woods. Beautiful trails can be found in almost every direction. It's been far too long since I have had the real experience. Evan is also an avid hiker and jumps at the chance to go anywhere in the woods, and for any increment of time. I was always the same exact way, and I'm starting to feel that way again. Getting my old life back in view certainly helped center my wayward thoughts.

76. Clarity

The weather outside is actually bearable for an adventure in the woods. I can tell that Evan is excited as he gets his backpack ready for the day. The two of us collectively have enough gear to get lost in the woods for over a week before it would even start to become uncomfortable. Being prepared for such a disaster is better than getting caught in one with nothing to depend on. I have always liked camping equipment for some reason – I think it's because of its efficiency. You can accomplish anything that you need to as long as you have the right tools with you. Not being limited in any way makes the experience perfect and ties everything together nicely. We'll only be taking a long hike today – nothing more, but I have everything with me anyways – standard protocol.

I have another whole setup of climbing gear which is still sitting in a closet at my mother's house. I didn't want to risk any of it getting stolen from my room, and didn't feel as though I needed it in my closet for any immediate reason. I have collected some of the best quality pieces over the years and have everything necessary to launch a fully fledged climb against any rock face there is. I love to climb, and hope to get back out there as soon as spring hits. It's then that I feel the most free.

Evan and I head out toward a trail that borders the edge of his backyard. For a half mile or so we will have to fight through thick brush before we finally meet up with a more frequently traveled trail which we will then change course onto. We have done this hike before so we know our way perfectly, but it has been so long that it has the excitement of being just like that very first time. Some areas of the trail look exactly how I remember, but strangely very different all at the same time. It's as if I notice the aged state of everything that used to look so bright and new. The trees are showing more wear than they used to as time ticks by and continues to eat away at them. The elements have shown their force by uprooting some vegetation that used to be firmly grasping the earth. The trail still remains the same though, winding its way through the forest and overcoming whatever obstacles cross its path. Small man made bridges have been put into place wherever a small stream cuts through the soil beneath. Other than help in these few places, everything else to be seen, found, or heard is completely natural.

After about two hours of steady pace we come to a lean-to that is frequented by many hikers. It's a popular destination, as they usually are, for people who are performing through-hikes and traveling across state borders for months on end. This has always been one of my long term goals. I don't think that there is anything else in the world would have such a profound effect on my mental state. The freedom that comes with it all is enough to clear my head completely, and it's the closest that I can get to the feeling of shooting up.

This particular lean-to resembles more of an abandoned cabin than a normal run of the mill lean-to. It is completely closed in and actually has a wooden hinged door that closes. The floor is constructed of large, rough wooden slats and there is even a built in table in one corner. A tradition that we apparently started, and always continued to maintain, was the constant supply of candles. There are a few designated places that have been setup with metal trays to burn candles on. Sometimes weeks would pass where nobody would visit the lean-to – things would be exactly as we left them. For some reason one day we decided to always keep the metal trays stocked with a fresh candle whenever we left the lean-to. Other hikers would visit the lean-to and word started to travel quickly as we noticed new candles being left on the trays. Currently there are about fifteen different candles on each of the two trays in the lean-to. They are all different shapes, sizes, and scents, and have been left here by many different people who have passed through during their travels. It's one of the coolest things I have ever been a part of.

Sitting inside on the hard rough flooring brought back memories of many different evenings. Some of them were extremely cold and the wind would make the entire lean-to creak throughout the night. One time we could hear wolves walking around outside and sniffing at the walls. There have been so many amazing experiences spent out here. It's too bad that we aren't staying the night. Evan is rearranging things in his backpack just like it's any other normal day out here. I am in a state of awe with how it all makes me feel – I guess it has just been too long.

We start getting ready for the next leg of the hike which will circle us around back to the lean-to in about three hours. It's the longest stretch of the journey, but ends back here which gives you something to look forward to. A large formation of rocks is at the peak of the hike – no matter what, it always looks the same. Its massiveness alone subsequently makes it untouchable to anything. Even the elements themselves don't seem to affect it. It's breathtaking to me every time I see it. The formation also marks the half-way point for the hike back to the lean-to. There are so many things out here that would never be seen if you didn't seek them out. I've always been a little too curious of my surroundings to not go take a look.

I feel cleaner out here in the woods – it always makes me feel that way. The outside world seems dirty and dingy in comparison. Here I am surrounded by life teeming in every direction. There's no better way to spend your time. It humbles me in many ways. I am a different person when I'm here – this is the only time that I feel this way. I need to do this for the rest of my life every single day. That needs to be my ultimate goal.

After hiking through the forest with Evan for a solid five hours I come to a realization that almost knocks me off of my feet. I haven't thought about heroin since we broke the tree line at the edge of his yard. I haven't had one thought about using. I haven't had even a twinge of a craving – nothing. My addicted mind has finally taken a vacation. That hasn't happened in over two years. I haven't had a single moment of peace from my drug riddled thoughts while in a conscious state. Sometimes my mind would poison my unconscious thoughts as well. This is monumental.

Evan is staring at me, as I suddenly realize that I have stopped moving completely, and am leaning up against a tree. My mind has never been this clear, or it has been so long since it has that I didn't remember what it felt like. Still shocked by this new revelation I slowly start to walk away from the tree – Evan still staring at me intently.

"It's ok man….really good thoughts…let's go." I pat him on the shoulder smiling and lead the way back down the trail.

77. Hope

E van is driving me home, and the thoughts return to my head occupying the spaces that they always used to. At least I know that I can deal with them, and I know how to make them go away. I have to stay focused and get to higher ground as quickly as possible. It's the only chance that I have to save myself for good. I have today's memories to help get me through the rough times in my head. I'm building a small arsenal of experiences to use in my defense. So far I like the direction that everything is going in.

Evan has been smiling ever since we got back to his house from the hike, he doesn't talk about anything in particular or offer a reason for his amusement, but I think he realizes that I had an epiphany back on the trail. I never fully understood before how much my sadness affected the people around me. Today I think I finally got it by seeing the look on his face during my "change". I stifle back the pain that is returning in full force – at least for the ride back to my room. It seems to be the appropriate thing to do.

Its dark outside already and there is a small group of people hovering around the front door to my building. Evan drops me off at the curb in front and I tell him that I'll get a hold of him soon. I walk past the congregation and head up to my room with my sleeping bag and backpack. Everything inside is untouched and exactly the way I left it – my little room waiting for me to return, and brutally reminding me of real life. I try to think about the small animal prints that I saw in the light snow covered ground in the woods. I can smell the air again in my mind and I forget about my tiny box of a room for a minute. Maybe I should just go through life with my eyes sealed shut – following scenery that I paint in my mind. Ignorance is indeed bliss, and I don't think that bothers me anymore. Not having to actually see the world's ugliness would help me to facilitate a state of happiness, and even perhaps sustain it. Being blind certainly has its advantages.

I gather up my three dirty dishes and random utensils from the other day when my brother was here and head to the kitchen to wash them in the sink. Surprisingly there is a communal bottle of dish soap that never seems to get stolen from the kitchen. It's pretty much the only thing in there that doesn't need to be bolted down. I find it odd that out of everything else – the dish soap is safe to be as vulnerable as possible. I'm not sure why anybody would really want to steal it, but usually these kinds of people don't ever need much of a reason. Either way it makes me happy, because that's one less thing that I have to worry about having. I'll gladly use the one that is there and return it when I'm done without question. Maybe that's why nobody steals it – we all want it to be there when we need it. Strange how things work sometimes.

The floor is relatively quiet for the most part, which I find to be a bit surprising. Usually it's only quiet when the cops are here – for whatever reason. Mostly its domestic disturbance or drug related when they do get called here. The couple downstairs will be tearing each others heads off in a drunken rage and the entire building goes quiet so they can all listen in on the argument. Everybody wants to know the exact details of what is going on. It provides some sort of rush for them – they live for it. They have to have the answers about everyone who lives in the building. Who works where, and what kinds of problems that person faces every day. This one got arrested for that, this one beat up that girl, this one has five kids in another state. The shit talk is always flying around and bouncing off of the crumby walls. I stay out of it all. I fly under the radar and do whatever I can to keep myself off of the grid. Polite when addressed, and otherwise invisible. So far it has been working perfectly, and I can't see any other way to do it.

Hope

My dishes are clean and I still haven't had the displeasure of running into anyone – I'll take this rare gift. I return to my room safely and lock the door behind me as always. I'm finally back in my little dungeon – and with clean dishes. My duties for the night are finished, and I don't even have to work today. I hit play on the boom box and pull out a small joint that Evan insisted I take with me – I barely put up an argument. I light it up and take a hit, then settle myself onto the futon with an empty notebook and a pen.

It has been a long time since I really sat down and wrote anything, but things are slowly changing now so it seems so natural to me. I had a slew of peaceful thoughts while I was in the woods today, and I want to get a few of them down before they are lost forever. I take another hit from the joint and start writing furiously on the first white lined sheet of paper I find. My hand is moving with a swiftness I have never witnessed before, and my thoughts are gushing down my arm screaming to stain the paper with black figures. I don't even see what I am writing, nor do I understand it for the most part, but it flows out of me nonetheless. I have once again conquered my tainted thoughts and pushed heroin as far away from me as possible. I snap at myself to not think about it, and continue writing in tongues.

My hand is killing me, and this is the first time that I have noticed. I'm halfway through the empty notebook as I turn to a fresh page. The last complete thought formulates in my head and as I write it down the pen runs out of ink. I stare at the paper in a daze. My cycle has finally been broken and I thumb back through the stack of pages that I have already completed. They are filled up on both sides with sentence after sentence of black ink. I notice some of the words as I flip back through the littered pages. I have managed to explain my exact feelings in perfect detail on the papers in front of me. Wild descriptions of moments on the trail are woven in and out of each paragraph which seems to be in no discernible order. A collection of thoughts spilled out onto paper. It was a perfect exercise and exactly the outlet that I needed. I have made great strides today in my recovery, and have felt things that I thought were lost forever. I have seen my first real glimmer of hope. I stare at the notebook in amazement and wonder what is going to come next.

78.   Need

Nikki is starting to get on my nerves more and more lately. She keeps coming into the store during my shifts and begging me to come back to her. I'm stuck between knowing what I should do – which is to stay away – and what my mind pushes me toward subconsciously. She's another one of my addictions that I find very hard to avoid. Even when she is standing in front of me at the store going on and on about irrelevant shit I can't help feeling the urge to wrap my arms around her and take her away. I have to tell myself over and over again that we don't work well together, and quite possibly never will. We aren't good for each other the way that we used to think we would be. We used to think that being together would ultimately help to keep us both clean. That notion has proven itself to be wrong many times over throughout the last year. We've tried and tried and tried, but failed miserably every single time, and almost instantly. I can never go back that way no matter how much I would love it to.

She finally agrees to leave and let me finish my shift, but under the condition that I head right over to her place after work tonight. Things have been good for me the past few days, because I haven't really had to deal with much. I have just recently started to get used to the new routines I have created for myself, and have finally found some creative ways to handle the negative thoughts that sometimes overwhelm my mind. I wasn't expecting the sudden blow out on her end, but I suppose that's my own blindness showing itself. I should have known that she wouldn't keep quiet forever, and as soon as she had nowhere better to turn – I'd be on the menu. I'm going to swing by her place simply to appease her tonight, but I'm going to explain to her that we cannot go back to the way things used to be. I have my shit together for the first time in a couple of years, and I'm still nowhere near getting myself out of the woods yet. She needs to deal with whatever bullshit keeps throwing her off course, and try to get a grip on herself again. I have to somehow make my motives clear when I arrive, or else she'll just use whatever weakness that she can to get under my skin, and when it comes to weaknesses – she knows them all. I just hope that I can stand my ground long enough to get my point across before she clouds me with whatever illusion she decides to spin up. She can snowball me so easily sometimes, it's like my IQ drops to six when I'm around her. I start thinking with all of the wrong organs, and my entire defense system quivers and falls to the ground. There are some things in this world that I am physically incapable of finding enough strength to battle. I eventually give up and throw in the towel. I can't let that happen tonight.

I start cleaning the store up at about 11:30pm, giving myself enough time to run the mop through it quickly. I hate this part of the job, but they consider it very important, so I pretty much have no choice but to do it. The mop bucket is disgusting and looks like it has been here since the beginning of time. The mop itself is also extremely used and stained black throughout. I doubt that it even cleans anything anymore because it obviously holds more dirt than what is actually on the floor. I don't bother lobbying for a new one though – if they think that it looks clean in the morning – that's all that matters. I guess there's no reason to fix something that isn't broken – even if it is actually broken.

After the store appears to be spic and span I grab myself a pack of smokes and get ready to lock the doors as I leave. I'm not anticipating a good time at Nikki's tonight, I have a feeling we are just going to go back and forth fighting until one of us completely loses it. Most likely it will be her who cracks first; I have a pretty long fuse. The walk to the apartment is pretty much the same distance that I used to travel on foot when I was staying there and working at the grocery store. The only difference is that I am coming from another direction. I should be there in about ten minutes give or take a few.

On the way over my thoughts are filled with blurbs that I desperately want to remember until I have an opportunity to write them down. I have been inundated with ideas lately that might not ever take shape in any real tangible form, but I want them to be recorded somehow nonetheless. It's a new way of thinking for me as I feel like my mind is under my control again, and not clouded by incessant cravings for heroin. I still continue to struggle with the flare ups, but don't even find myself reaching for the bottle anymore to deal with them. I have definitely turned a corner in the right direction, and constantly remind myself to not question it – just let it ride.

Nikki meets me at the door already with a drink in her hand, which I didn't anticipate. She was never a big drinker really, so I'm surprised that she even took it upon herself to have alcohol readily available. Must be some knew kind of behavior that I just haven't seen yet. She decides to take a more hospitable approach with me and gives me a kiss as I walk in the front door – once again catching me off guard. I forgot how good she was at manipulating people – she's doing it to me right now. I can't let it work – I must stand my ground.

"We can't get back together." I say to her in the sternest voice I can muster. Her smile drops to an immediate frown and she starts walking toward me while taking her top off. She has nothing on underneath, and has clearly had lots of time to prepare herself for this meeting. She has already planned each precise step of this process, and is ready for every turn it might take. I have not come as prepared, and will give in at any moment – I can feel it.

Quickly scanning the room I don't see any drug paraphernalia laying around, which calms my nerves ever so slightly. At least I'm not going to have to deal with that tonight – yet. I decide that ruling out the possibilities would be stupid and leave me even more vulnerable that I already am. Stand my ground.

Before I know it she is wrapped around me wearing nothing but a pair of skimpy panties that can barely pass as an undergarment of any kind. They cover virtually nothing, and might as well not be there at all. I feel her warm skin against mine, and can't help myself but to touch her all over. It's been so long since I was with a woman and more specifically since I have been with her. She has made her way into my head, and is exploiting every dirty little thought that I have ever had. I pick her up and carry her over to the bed that I used to sleep in every night. I tear the covers off and throw them on the floor in an instant. This is a temptation that I cannot walk away from.

The two of us have wild sex all over the apartment for hours and hours until we finally find the strength to peel ourselves apart from each other. The sun is starting to come up outside, and I realize that neither of us have even spoken since I got there. Nikki gives me an understanding look, which I am immediately surprised about. I think she gets it, and perhaps she'll stop trying to get us back together – it's just not going to work. I throw my clothes on hastily and head out toward the street. That was a weird night, but I really don't have anything to complain about overall. My thoughts are consumed with sexual fantasies as I slowly make the walk across town to my tiny little room.

79. Slipping

The last few days have been uneventful for the most part. Nikki has kept away from me, only visiting me twice so far at the store, and for reasonable amounts of time. She hasn't brought up the topic of us getting back together again, but I suspect that I haven't heard the end of it yet. She looks at me a certain way like she wants to say something but then decides not to at the last minute. I'm not going to let myself get too excited yet in thinking that she actually has accepted things for what they are. At any moment that excitement could be taken away from me if she decides to go crazy, which isn't an unreasonable expectation. Coming from her, nothing is really much of a surprise anymore.

My brother is happy that I'm staying clean. I can tell the difference in his voice whenever I talk to him, and how he is when he visits. He seems to be a lot more relaxed now when we are together, probably because he isn't worried all the time that something is going to happen to me. I can tell that he's always still on his toes ready for whatever might come, but not with as much rigidity as before. The roller coaster ride of my previous life certainly took its toll on him, but he stuck right there with me whenever he could – better than anyone else even tried. Not that I fault anyone for that at all. I'm just forever going to be in debt to him – that's for sure.

It's a little after midnight and I am climbing the stairs to my room. My mind is wandering in a million different directions as it has been ever since the quick hike with Evan. I'm thinking about what thought I want to put into writing first when I get to my room – and then I see it. I am about to step onto a landing before I climb the next set of stairs, and I find myself frozen – stuck to the floor. In the corner of the landing – still in perfect shape – is a shiny new needle. The black lines running down the clear plastic tube are perfectly visible. My body reacts in shock and prevents me from doing anything. My mind goes blank to the outside world and becomes all consumed with thoughts of heroin. Every muscle in my body twitches with craving and sweat breaks out of the pores on my forehead. I force my hand to let go of the metal railing in order to move past the wayward needle. I can't take my eyes off of it. I want to fill it up and use it over and over again until the tip of the needle is too dull to pierce skin. My hand slowly moves up the railing and grasps onto the round pipe with unbearable force once again. I can feel my knuckles turning white. My vision becomes hazy and it feels like I'm going to go down. It feels like the walls are caving in on me and at any moment I will be buried in rubble. I finally turn and hold onto the railing with both hands. My breathing is labored and heavy, my heart is thrashing in my chest. I have to make it to my room. I continue to pull myself toward the next set of stairs and climb them slowly so as not to pass out. I fight the urge to turn my head and look back at it. I fight the urge to run to it. I fight every piece of motivation in my body and make my way to the top of the stairs. Through the door and down the hallway – I'm finally in my room again. I stumble to the futon and frantically find the bottle of vodka. I can't get enough alcohol in me fast enough, and then I start to relax all the while rocking back and forth on the edge of my mattress. That was the first time I have come into contact with anything directly related to heroin. I didn't anticipate what would happen if I ever did, but I would never have been prepared for that anyways. I focus all of my energy on getting it off of my mind and stare at the opposite wall of my room for hours. Nothing in my immediate vision ever changes, and if it does, I don't notice it. I stare and stare until I can't anymore, and then I fall asleep.

Something woke me up, but I have no idea what. I just know that there was a ruckus of some sort that worked its way into the dream I was having, and that it subsequently woke me up. That ruckus is gone now, so I have no idea what it might have been – I think that it was people outside though. I remember the voices being muffled in my dream, and hard to understand fully. I'm still at the end of the futon staring at the wall, just in a laying down position now. The drawing of a skeleton hanging from a rope has been peaking my interest in the last few days. I think the reason why I like it is because it looks very crudely drawn, but in fact it is extremely intricate and carefully thought out. Upon closer inspection you can see where the artist has actually included hairline cracks in each of the bones to add a more realistic tone to the subject. The rope that is tied around the skeleton's neck is also very detailed. You can see the individual strands of the rope all twisted together. This person really spent a lot of time on their creation. It's probably just what they consumed all of their free time with while they were here. Regardless I've taken quite the liking to it, and I'm going to miss it if I ever get a new place.

It's still very dark out and obviously not much time has passed since I came down from my freak out earlier and fell asleep. I'm guessing that it's around 3:00am. I'm feeling a lot better, but still find myself a bit jilted from the whole thing. I'm still clutching the bottle of vodka with my left hand. I pop the cap off and take another big hit. That should help me to sleep through the rest of the night, or at least that's what I'm hoping for.

80. Suspicion

My days have gotten darker. I do my best at all times to balance the thoughts in my head, but sometimes the bad ones win. They haven't gotten the best of me yet, and they don't bother me as much as they used to, but they certainly aren't going away anytime soon. The good thoughts are perfect, but I can't hold on to them all the time – no matter how hard I try. I just can't seem to get past this last leg of the process. I'm not using, which is the most important part, but I can't find a way to make things any easier than I already have. This way of life is foreign, and all such a mystery to me.

I see the addicts come in and out of the store all night long while I'm at work. They look like shit. They are always trying to scheme on free water, or whatever they can get their hands on. I understand this mentality all too well. They are constant reminders of how my life used to be, which is helpful, and not, all at the same time. I can't decide whether I hate them or love them. They are the epitome of what I understand – no matter how wrong it is. I envy them at times for being on the other side of the counter. I find myself staring off into space waiting for the time to pass. I find myself doing nothing at all.

Fighting a depression without drug use really wears a person out. It starts from the inside and slowly erodes its way through your body until you have no strength to do anything anymore. No motivation, no cares, nothing. There has got to be something more. There has to be another reason for performing all of these mindless tasks. There has to be life beyond life.

My skin burns with desire to use every time I think about heroin. I envision my body bright red and steaming with heat. I'll burst into flames at any moment if I can't get relief. My body will turn to dust and blow away as soon as the next customer opens the glass door at the front of the store. They can loot the place because I am the only one working, and now I'm gone. They'll eventually find my scorched remains in a small pile behind the register that I was standing at. There will be no way to identify me, so it will just be assumed that it was me. Someone will scoop up my ashes in a plastic bag and presumably carry me over to a funeral home. Either that or toss me in the dumpster – at that point who really gives a shit? It's not like I am going to care all that much, I won't even have the ability to. Some people are nuts about arrangements – I don't get it.

Another junkie walks in and buys a pack of smokes from me. The gas pumps outside are beeping and waiting for my authorization of the sale. Someone is filling up a giant plastic cup full of green slop from the slushy machine in the corner. My mind is racing around the store trying to catch up with the time that I lost while day dreaming. I might have been staring at this guy for five minutes – I'm not sure. I don't remember.

Evan called me about an hour ago and wants to hang out again tonight. I agreed, reluctantly. For some reason I just can't seem to make myself happy about anything. I'm hoping that perhaps another night away from my little room will be therapeutic and help in some way. I anticipate that it's not going to make that much of a difference though. I anticipate that it actually might make things worse, because Evan is still under the impression that I'm in a really good place mentally. He asked me what was wrong when we spoke on the phone, apparently he could tell by my voice. I told him nothing, and tried to sound a bit more enthusiastic – I don't think that I did a very good job.

I have three hours left before it's time to lock this place up and hit the road. I'm going to go insane if I can't find a faster way to make this time pass. I pull out a blank sheet of paper and start doodling on it with a pen – drawing random shapes and scribbles all over the place. I just want to cover the entire thing with black ink and make it disappear. Another customer walks in and I'm forced to put the pen down. At least it's something to do for a minute. Another pack of smokes leaves the store, that's all anyone ever buys here. The profit that comes in from cigarettes alone could keep this store running – I'm convinced. I steal my packs from here – fuck that. Tick them off of the inventory list every night, and nobody is the wiser. They won't miss my five bucks.

I notice that some asshole has spilled an entire coffee on the floor by the beverage station. The coffee is dripping down the counter and hitting every single thing in its path. I didn't see it happen, or see which asshole did it, but now I have to clean it up. This pisses me off on principle – I don't like cleaning up some other idiot's mess. It seems so wrong to me, like I'm their personal servant. "Sure dump your shit all over the floor sir – I'll just clean it up for you." I should announce that to each person that walks in the door, because ultimately it's true. Either that or just get it printed on a gigantic sandwich board sign that I can wear all day long – just so that there's no confusion.

I grab the spray bottle and paper towels from behind the counter and head out to the mess. Begrudgingly I start slopping up the coffee and try to get it cleaned up as quickly as I can. I want to go back to the safety of my counter. I want to continue working on my doodle page masterpiece. I have priorities. The phone rings as I'm heading back to the counter. I answer it just in time – It's Evan.

"Hey man…ummmm….so we're still on for later?" He asks me in a strange voice.

"Yeah" I answer wearily.

"Ok……I was just checking….I'll see you at 12." He hangs up the phone.

That was weird. That was really weird. I have no idea why he would have called me to check if we were still on for later. He doesn't do that, and I don't usually change my plans – he knows this. There was motivation behind that phone call that I can't seem to put my finger on. I don't like it. I don't like it at all actually. My mind is going off on a thousand different tangents – every one of them just as bad if not worse than the last. I have two more agonizing hours to sit here and speculate. It's going to drive me completely insane, and I can't wait for him to get here so that I can put whatever it is to rest. Whatever outlandish thing he is thinking – I need to know what it is. I need to know what weird thing he has cooked up in his head, and I sincerely hope that my instincts are wrong, otherwise – I already know what it is.

81. Acting

Evan picks me up, and I immediately want to know what's up. He seems to be hiding it well so far as we drive down the dark road in silence. The anxiety from his last phone call has disappeared from his voice, but that doesn't fool me. He wanted to ask me something during that call, but chickened out. He wanted to bring something up, but then decided not to. He wanted another hit. I know that's what he was yearning for. I recognized the desperation in his voice when he started talking; I just told myself that I was wrong. Now that I can see him in person though – I'm convinced that's what it was. He was struggling with bringing it up because he doesn't want to hinder my progress. He knows that it's wrong to do anything that would push me back into the hands of that terrible drug, but his own craving is getting the best of him. I'm not going to bring it up unless he does, just in case I'm wrong.

The ride to his house seems just as normal as any other time. I am looking forward to getting away from my room, and I once again have tomorrow off. These are the highlights of my life now I guess – taking a one day vacation from work two towns away and walking through the woods, providing the weather can hold up. I guess I really shouldn't be complaining about it, I just wish that there was something more than this, eventually there has to be, I'm just going to keep telling myself that.

The trees seem very dark tonight as we make our way down the winding back roads toward his house. There is something especially eerie about them tonight, but I can't quite figure it out. It might be due to the fact that the moon is almost full and the light from it is casting a blue haze on everything it touches. It makes me feel like something bad is about to happen, like when you get that lump in the pit of your stomach for no reason. I try not to think about it, and focus on getting back down into the basement.

Evan immediately pulls out the bong – just like last time. I certainly have no complaints, especially with how weird the night has been already. Its times like these that freak me out the most – when you just really have no idea what is going on. I hate that feeling. I like to be as ready as I can be for disaster, especially if it is staring me square in the face. I give Evan a questioning look, giving him a chance to speak on it, but he declines and breaks eye contact with me quickly. I think that I caught him off guard. I don't think that he expected me to know as much as I know. I'm not easily fooled when it comes to shit like this, and he of all people should know that, but when you are up to no good sometimes you don't think as clearly as you normally do.

I take a giant hit off of the bong and lean back against the wall next to his bed. I start to flow with the music as always and clear my head of any negative thoughts in the process. Evan is still pretending that everything is perfect, so I decide to just go along with the charade. He starts telling me about things at work, which I actually do find quite interesting. Evan's job as a chef is something that I actually wouldn't mind doing for a living. I always like listening to whatever he had to make for the day; usually the meals are very involved. I like the fact that they use so many different resources and ingredients to make their creations. I used to find recipes that were very involved and looked good, just to try them out on my own, back when I actually had use of a halfway stocked kitchen.

Evan begins telling me about this large pasta dish that he had to make for a banquet earlier tonight. Some of his help dropped the ball on some things causing Evan to improvise, which he is usually very good at doing. When you get put in the position of needing to make fast accurate decisions all the time you tend to get pretty good at it. Evan can definitely think on his feet, but only when its food related. In normal real world situations he tends to be a bit slow actually, which I have always found to be quite amusing. This is precisely why he is dancing around me with the topic of heroin. He knows that he shouldn't bring it up to me, but he has nobody else to turn to about it. No other way that he can think of to get another hit. He's certainly not going to go out and find the shit on his own, and he's not even going to give himself his own shot – I always do it for him. Everything about this drug freaks Evan out, except for the feeling that it provides when you are on it. He needs me in order to feel it again. He's only used twice in the past four months or so, but it still freaks me out that he's itching to do it again. That's still one more chance closer to getting hooked – all it takes is one special time.

I decide to call it an early night and get my sleeping bag ready. Evan starts climbing into bed as well, he's probably glad that I haven't tried pushing my suspicion any further than the strange look I gave him a few minutes ago. Eager to get some sleep and perhaps take a hike tomorrow, I wrap myself up in the sleeping bag and roll over onto my side. My own terrible drug ridden thoughts have somehow eluded me at the moment, and I anticipate a nice peaceful sleep. I close my eyes and welcome the darkness that surrounds me. I want to be well rested for tomorrow.

82. Honesty

The morning is normal as we pack up our gear. We are going to take the same hike that we did last week, using the lean-to as a stopping point. Evan looks eager to get outside as we make our way upstairs to leave. I can tell that there is still something on his mind that he is struggling to bring up, but he's acting like everything is normal. I'd almost be fooled if I didn't fully understand what I was dealing with. This is easily a subject that I can actually call myself an expert on. I understand the motivation.

The woods are as marvelous as ever, but I still can't seem to grasp my hands around the happiness I felt last week. The episode at my building the other night really drained me and has pushed me into a slump of sorts. I'm in a fragile state right now when it comes to dealing with my addiction. Sleep hasn't been easy back at my room. I have been trying to stay away from the alcohol as much as possible, but I haven't had a night without it since. Maybe I need some more time out here. I should try to get a few consecutive days off at work and plan an actual hike that will last a few nights. Maybe that will help my happiness to return and keep my mind off of the past. I'll do anything at this point. Especially considering how dull my life has gotten since I've been clean. I have to do something to curve my thoughts or I am just going to end up failing again.

It's a little colder out today than it was last week. My face is going to be numb by the time we reach the lean-to, but it will warm up quickly once we get inside. The wind is swirling through the trees creating a sound that closely resembles a whistle, but not quite as shrill. It adds to the overwhelmingly vacant undertone of the woods today. Evidence of the animals who call this place home can be found with careful observation. Even the birds are especially quite today leaving the illusion that

Evan and I are all alone amongst the trees. Continuing along the trail I wait for the freedom like feeling to take over my thoughts, but it never seems to fully engage. I'm still anticipating a conversation with Evan, which seems to be completely consuming my thoughts. I keep moving in the correct direction hoping that at any moment he'll bring up whatever it is he wants to talk about, just to get it over with.

We approach the lean-to in silence and I can feel that the change is about to take place. Once inside I set down my backpack and look straight into Evan's eyes. This takes him off guard for a minute, which is what I was hoping for.

"What's on your mind?" I ask him.

"Nothing." He replies.

"Bullshit. You've been avoiding something ever since last night when you called me at the store, and I think I already know what it is." Evan looks around the lean-to as if he is checking to make sure that nobody else is within earshot. I try not to smile at this gesture – it must just be instinctual.

"I want another hit. I want to feel it again. Fuck….I shouldn't have said anything."

My body quickly shakes with a pulse of heat that surges through my veins. I brush it off and gather my thoughts.

"No. You can't just have another hit whenever you want, and I can't be around that shit anymore. It's not like smoking a cigarette – you're playing Russian roulette with this shit man. Haven't I set enough of an example?" I say to him flustered.

"I know, I know, but I just thought one more time wouldn't hurt anything, just like the last time."

"Of course it will hurt something – every single time that you use you get one step closer to being sucked in – you have to get it out of your head. Smoke some weed and be happy, you don't want that shit anywhere near you – trust me." I pick my backpack up and head toward the door.

"Where are you going?" Evan asks in a worried tone.

"Back on the trail. We need to keep moving." I answer and step back out into the cold.

Evan follows behind me for a minute or so before he catches up to my pace. I'm moving with significant speed out of sheer frustration caused by the conversation I was dreading. I didn't want to be right in my speculation. I didn't want that to actually be what was on his mind. I didn't want to believe that he would entertain using again, and furthermore bring it up to me knowing that I have been clean for two months now. As a friend he should have known better than to plant that seed in my head. I'm in such a fragile state as it is – this is just going to eat away at me along with everything else. No matter where I turn or what I do, I just can't seem to get away from this drug.

I decide to not bring it up again, providing that he doesn't, which I can't guarantee. Evan doesn't act like he wants to talk about it, so I think that I might be safe for now. I'm still very uneasy about the entire situation, and can't seem to get my mind off of it, but I'm desperately trying to do whatever I can to accomplish just that.

Reaching the giant rock formation helped more than I expected. There's something about its overall power that puts things into perspective for me. I am awed by its beauty, and by the power that nature can have at any given moment. The balance that must occur in order for things like this to sustain themselves is beyond any logical thought process. A small group of hikers approach from the opposite direction and snaps me out of my trance like state. Evan and I nod our heads at them and continue on our loop.

After a few more hours we manage to make our way back to Evan's house. Relaxing in the basement seemed like a great idea, but Evan is still a bit jilted about the conversation we had in the lean-to. I'm still avoiding it like the plague. I take a few hits off of the bong and announce that he should bring me back to my room for the night. I need to collect my thoughts before going back to work tomorrow. I need Evan to get these thoughts out of his head, and me being in his presence doesn't help I'm sure. Without hesitation Evan rounds up the essentials and heads up the stairs – I eagerly follow behind him.

The car ride back to my room was quiet for the most part, but not awkward really. We clearly both avoided continuing the conversation in the woods; at least he's just as uncomfortable about it as I am on some level. Back in my room once again it feels like a gigantic weight has been lifted off of my chest. I can't figure out how to deal with this yet, and really needed to be alone again. I'm chain smoking and will need a new pack soon if I continue at this rate. I'm nervous that I am going to be up all night stressing about everything. It's going to be even harder to curve my cravings knowing that Evan is just waiting for me to pull the trigger on using. I eye my bottle of vodka which I replaced the other night with a new one. It's about half full and should get me through the night without too much trouble. Things can't stay this way though. I can't keep drowning myself in alcohol in order to deal with the addiction itself. Before I know it I'm going to be physically addicted to that too which will be one more thing to deal with avoiding. There's no way I can let that happen or else I'll be screwed on so many levels. I'll pretend that Evan isn't itching to use, and that everything is just as it was before I went there. Something has got to give.

83. Losing

Work is starting to feel as it always did – like shit. I don't want to be here. I don't want to come here. I don't want to ever even think about it. I'm turning into everything that I hate. I'm turning into just another robot that wanders the earth constantly in search of nothing. I'm so depressed by this thought that I find it hard to move my limbs. My lips hang stupidly from my face and are completely out of my control. I have become a zombie. The familiar beep,beep,beep noise constantly loops through my brain as each "number" approaches the counter. I'm exactly where I was before I started using. Nothing has changed beyond my addiction. Now I get to be miserable all of the time like usual, and fight something more powerful than myself on top of it. There has to be a way to break this cycle. Whatever it is – I desperately need to find it, because I'm not sure how much longer I can go on like this. Evan's recent confession has my head spinning with ideas. I could have a fix within the next two hours if need be. The temptation has grown into a real tangible thing that I carry around with me all day. I have no idea how to get rid of it, and am not convinced if I will ever succeed in doing so.

I ring up another "number" and watch the glass door slowly close behind them. There's only one other person in the store at the moment – they're the type of person that can't decide what kind of drink to buy so they stare at the coolers in wonder for minutes on end. I love watching them because they change their minds as fast as they decide on something. One lady picked up six different drinks and put them back one by one before finally deciding on buying the seventh. It's unbelievable the time that people will spend on the most irrelevant decisions. All I can surmise is that these people must have really boring lives that require no real thoughts to sustain. This is the exact type of person I want to avoid becoming. I would rather die.

The phone rings, which seems a lot louder than usual, and I tear the counter apart looking for the cordless handset. It gets left in the strangest places sometimes. I find it shoved into a cubby under the register and answer it just in time. It's Nikki.

"We need to talk." She says to me right away.

"Ok.......what?" I ask somewhat annoyed at her tone. There's a silence on the other end of the phone as I listen to her slow breathing. It's then that I realize she's going to tell me something important. I'm not prepared for whatever it is and can feel my jaw tighten with anticipation.

"I'm pregnant."

I can barely continue to stand. My knees almost buckle as my head tries to understand the words that just came out of the receiver. A million thoughts hit me all at once and at first it's too much to handle. Thoughts of fatherhood, and what that will ultimately look like. Thoughts of how important my role would be in this person's life. Fear of not being ready, especially in my current state. Thoughts of how it even happened. I can't process a single thing fully before the next one takes over my thinking. I had forgotten that the phone was still up to my ear until Nikki spoke again.

"I'm having an abortion."

All of the thoughts I had just had were suddenly flipped around in an instant. A world of ideas completely backwards now and irrelevant. Before I could even start to comprehend the first piece of information I was presented with another impossibility. My brain feels like it has been put into a giant metal vice and a thousand people are cranking the handle tighter and tighter. I open my mouth to scream – but nothing comes out. I don't even know where to begin. So I do what comes to mind first and hurl the phone at the wall on the opposite side of the store. It hits hard and explodes into a million pieces all over the floor. The person that was so intently looking for a drink jumps a foot and leaves hastily. I can't believe what I just heard, and once again find myself glued to the floor unable to move, only standing this time.

How could all of this be happening? What am I going to do? I need to talk to her again as soon as I regain my composure. She can't do this to me. I will do whatever needs to be done to try and change her mind, but I've already been through a situation just like this in the past, and I'm not doing it again. As afraid as I may be I can't run away from this, and for some reason I especially can't this time. Things feel different now, and I need to be responsible for my actions as much as possible. I can't let her just make that decision without hearing me out first. Two more "numbers" walk into the store and I slowly go back to my spot behind the register. Everything feels numb as I hand them their smokes and throw cash in the tray. Tingling sensations travel through my limbs with every movement that I make. I'm in full-on zombie mode now. The people will come and go as they please just like any normal night, as I slowly wither away to nothing inside. My chest will continue to burn with anger and sorrow as I authorize gasoline sales and mop the white tiled floor. It will be a miracle if I make it back to my room tonight – it seems so far away. I feel like if I started walking to it right now that I wouldn't get there until the early morning hours. The world itself has been pushed away from me in my mind. I can reach out with my hands, but the illusion gets me every time as I grasp at nothing for hours on end. Somewhere in between the spaces there lies an answer – I just have to keep searching for it.

84. Dealing

I'm trying very hard not to destroy anything as I sit in my room. I'm staring at the walls trying very hard not to think about anything either. Every thought I have just immediately leads me to disaster. I can't think about Evan at all or my entire body shakes with unbearable cravings – knowing that he is sitting there ready at any moment to get a fix is just about killing me. If only he understood the magnitude of that tiny little conversation we had in the lean-to. It takes every single ounce of energy that I have left in order to prevent me from calling him. If heroin was within eyesight right now – I'd use it. I'd throw all of my progress away without even thinking twice. This is a really bad sign – obviously I'm wearing down. I don't know what to do.

Nikki and I have had numerous fights about the pregnancy, and so far she has not budged one bit on her decision. She is being completely unreasonable and will simply not listen to my argument on the matter. I can't bear to think of her getting an abortion, and I have no logical reason why. Oddly enough I think that I can handle being a father. I think that on many levels it's exactly what I need to be doing right now. I feel that raising my own child would straighten me out faster than any other rehabilitation method. Whenever I think about it an overwhelming sense of joy fills my entire body. It's a feeling that I have never felt before, and it's really good.

No matter what I say to her though she will not waver. She is standing her ground like a giant redwood tree that has lived to be one hundred and fifty years old. She feels that it would be a horrible environment for the child between her medical issues and my irresponsibility. Having one child that she already can't see doesn't help things either. She throws that in my face as well, as if the two things are related somehow. I even told her that I would take the kid once she has it and she can sign her rights away if she wants. Still no.

I have no idea what to do. I wait every couple of hours and then I call her again just to have everything that I am going to say fall on deaf ears. I can't get her to see my side at all, and she openly thinks that I'm nuts. She thinks that I am out of my mind to think that I can take care of a newborn baby on my own. She's the one that's nuts though.

My hands are tied, which is driving me completely insane. I can't stand that she has power over this situation and ultimately can do whatever she wants regardless of my wishes. I don't do very well in situations like these, where I can't even have any input that will make a difference. I would at least like a vote – something. Nothing, nothing, nothing is all I get. As usual.

I'm trying very hard not to destroy anything. I look at each item in my room and imagine it exploding in slow motion. I see each little particle fly off into the air immediately following the blast. The small fragments get farther and farther apart from each other until they finally land on the floor or collide into a nearby wall. Throwing one of the empty vodka bottles would give me immense satisfaction. Almost like the cordless phone at work the other night when I first learned this horrific news. That thing morphed into a thousand pieces. I was actually surprised at how broken it was when I went and cleaned it all up. I left a note for the manager saying that I had no idea where the cordless phone was, and couldn't find it all night. Hopefully that puts me in the clear, and I don't see how anyone will possibly be able to figure out what actually happened to it. I swept all of the pieces up into a plastic bag and threw it in a random dumpster on my walk home from work.

I don't remember anything from my walk home and have lost all concept of time. I'm not even sure how long I have been sitting here in my room staring at random objects. I think that I have missed work though – one shift at least, maybe two. I need to check on that and keep shit going there, but I just can't face the outside yet. I can't go talk to people or even look at them yet. I can't even fake it. I'm afraid that I will either snap completely and go crazy on someone, or have a full on mental break down right there in the middle of the store. For now I am going to stay here where it's safe and eventually I'll make my way back out into the real world. There will come a time when I don't have a choice, so I'll just wait until then.

There's a knock on my door. What? Now what? I can't take any surprises right now. It takes me a minute or so to walk the three feet from the mattress to the door. I look through the tiny peep hole. It's my brother. Fuck. He's going to know that something is wrong – immediately, and I can't have that conversation with him yet. I also have to make sure he doesn't think that I am using again, because that would be even worse – especially because it's not true. I take a deep breath and open the door.

"Hey, what's up with you man?" My brother asks immediately.

"Nikki and I got into a fight….again. That's all." I answer in my most convincing voice. He looks at me with a hint of skepticism, but then I can tell that he believes me. Dodged a bullet there – so far that is.

"I stopped by the store because I thought you'd be working. Adam asked me where you were, so I lied and told them you were sick which was why I was stopping in. I think they bought it – they didn't seem upset or anything like that. You need to call them though if you're not going to make it in bro."

"Thanks man, I know. I couldn't remember if I was working or not and then time just got the best of me. Until you brought it up I hadn't even thought about it for a few hours. I had every intention of running downstairs and calling from the payphone. Seriously thanks for doing that though. This shit with Nikki and I is really getting to me." I look around the room embarrassed at the state of things. It looks like I haven't left here in weeks, but really it has only been a couple of days. My brother plops himself down on the edge of the mattress and lights up a smoke. He pulls out a small bag of green stuff and tosses it to me with some rolling papers. Getting a little buzz right now is exactly what I need – I lay everything out on the trunk and get to work immediately.

I hand the freshly rolled joint to my brother and he lights it up without hesitation. He seems a bit stressed out as well, but he usually handles things better than I do. I hide in the corner somewhere waiting for it all to pass, while he just deals with everything head on. I've never understood his process, but it always works out well in the long run. It's good to have him here today, and I wish that I could tell him what's going on, but I can't bring myself to talk about it yet. Not with anyone.

My brother reaches over and pops a tape in the boom box that he just pulled out of his hoodie. It's a staple album – usually what we listen to when we are taking a ride in his car. The familiar instruments calm my nerves a little, and for the first time in days I feel somewhat sane. He is trying not to grill me on the Nikki subject. At first I thought that he brushed it off as just another bullshit fight between the two of us, but I think that he's figured out there's something more to it than that. He'll keep it to himself though unless I give him a reason to do otherwise. I can't let my guard down anymore than I already have while he's here. I need time to sort this all out before I can have an actual conversation about it with anyone – especially my brother.

He looks like he's going to hang out for a bit, so I reach over and crank the boom box up. My brother passes me the joint once again, and the two of us zone out to the music while filling my room with smoke.

85. Done

I've gone over everything in my head a thousand times. Think, think, think is all I do, and no matter what I keep ending up in the same place. With everything piling up on top of each other, I can't seem to get the inevitable out of my head. I know that I shouldn't do it, but I don't think that I can resist any longer. I think that I have to do it, or at least that is what I have convinced myself. My vile mind has decided to taint every thought I have with the same thing. Heroin. Heroin. Heroin. I can feel it calling me from around every corner. It's all I see in my vision no matter where I look. The process runs through my mind on a constant loop all day, and all night long. There's no way that I'm going to be able to stay away from it anymore. I have to have it. I have to feel it. I want it more than life itself, especially now. All I have to do is call Evan – that's it. That's how easy it will be to get this process started.

I have returned to work, but it's not really me who shows up for my shift. It's a mere shell of myself that I have robotically forced to walk in the front door of the store. I stand behind the counter and systematically hand people what they want while taking their money. Life spins out of control in front of me as I stare in a comatose state. I have nothing left inside of me to do it any other way. I'm sure that I'm not going to last too much longer here either, but for now I'm giving it my best shot.

I have started looking for another place to live – another room somewhere, because that's all that I'm able to afford at the moment. I have to get out of my current building though, it's too fucked up. The shit that goes on there makes me feel like I'm barely above homeless. The scum that go in and out of the front doors all night long are starting to give me the creeps, or at least make me feel like I'm just as bad as they are. My brother has a friend that lives in a large house which is setup in a similar

Done

fashion, but it's only a handful of people who live there, and things are quite different. He's going to check on availability for me, and hopefully I can make a move in the next week or so. It's just too depressing to walk home at night now. My destination is always a shithole, and filled with shithole people. My tolerance for such things is wearing down, a change has to occur.

The cordless phone still hasn't been replaced here yet. There is a backup corded phone in the back room, which I am on my way to right now. I have finally worked up the gall, and have made my final decision. All of this shit is tearing me apart from the inside out, and my breaking point has definitely been obliterated. Honestly I think that it happened a long time ago, but I was able to stand my ground for just a few more weeks. That time has passed though, and now I just don't give a fuck. I'm going to call Evan.

The phone rings and rings and rings, but nobody picks up. Fuck. I finally make the move and nobody is even there to answer. Typical. I slam the phone down and make my way back out to the counter slowly, hoping that nobody is there waiting to buy cigarettes. Nobody is there, and the store is empty. I can hear the clock ticking. It ticks so loud that my eardrums feel like they are going to explode. I would swear that someone was hitting a giant rock with a metal baseball bat with every second that passes. I can't believe that Evan wasn't home. Fuck.

I feel like running back to the phone again and ripping it off the wall. I feel like destroying it just like I did the cordless handset, but then I'll really have no way to get in touch with anyone, so I decide against it. Another asshole walks in and buys lottery tickets. I have no patience to deal with his indecisiveness and stand there blankly while he ponders which losing ticket to buy. What the fuck is wrong with these people? I am seconds from throwing them all at him when he finally asks for the last one and produces some cash. My teeth are clenched as I put the money in the drawer – I have to get out of here.

It's only been ten minutes when I find myself crawling back to the phone that is hanging on the wall. I can't stand it, and I have to try calling Evan again. Maybe he was in the bathroom and just didn't get to it in time. Maybe he was outside and he just got home. Either way, trying again won't hurt anything. I pick it up and dial his number with lighting speed. This time he answers on the third ring.

"Christ....don't you ever answer your phone?" I shout at him, and then realize how ridiculous I'm being. "Listen...I'm ready to do this. That thing we talked about the other day out in the woods....let's do it...one more time."

I hear silence on the other end of the phone as I wait for his response. Finally he breaks it.

"You're absolutely sure man?"

"Yes...100%. Can I take your car tomorrow?" I ask in a very desperate tone.

"Sure, but I want to come with you this time. I'll already be in town in the afternoon and can just swing by and pick you up. Then we can run up to my place right after."

"Fine...pick me up at my place when you're ready, I'll be there." I hang up the phone. I don't like this, but there's really no reason to argue with him. If he wants to take the drive down with me that badly – fuck it. I don't care at this point, at least not enough to stop him. It's probably a better idea anyways with the shape that I'm in. I'm even going to make him drive, that way there's less chance of anything stupid happening on the road. I can't believe that I'm actually going to do this.

A customer starts banging his fist on the counter, and I realize that I'm still standing in the back room staring at the hung up phone. I make my way back out to the counter and find myself grinning as I approach the irate "number". The dickwad that is standing there looks up at me in anger, but then suddenly changes his expression.

"Uh...can I get twenty bucks on pump.....three?" He asks me warily.

"Sure" I reply still grinning deeply. I toss the money in the register and hit the appropriate buttons on the archaic machine that controls the pumps. He steals one last quick glance at me and heads back out toward his car. I have obviously completely lost it, and it seems to be written all over my face. It will be a small miracle if I get out of this place tonight without getting myself arrested for annihilating some poor fucker who just happens to say the wrong thing to me. I fully understand why people snap now, because I'm teetering right on the edge of rational thought. I want so badly to hit fast forward and be sitting in Evan's basement cooking up a shot. I want the next twenty four hours to have already passed, and without any bullshit. I want to feel the rush again, and make all of the pain go away. I'm planning on doing just that, and can't wait to tear down anything that dares to stand in my way.

86. Hell

Last night was terrible. Completely horrendous, and almost unbearable. I should have known better than to make plans to score heroin and then sleep on it. I should have known what that would have done to me mentally. What's another night of suffering though? I've certainly been through enough in the past that last night seems quite tame in comparison. I'm still here this morning – burning with desire, but still here nonetheless. I can do this.

I've parked myself up against the trunk while sitting on the mattress. I haven't moved from this position in hours, and don't currently plan to. I'm waiting for the knock on my door, which I have left unlocked so that Evan can just walk in when he arrives. I don't want anything to get in the way, or hinder this plan in any manner. My fix is still very far away, and I need to stay focused in order to get my hands on it. An empty bottle of vodka stares at me from where it's laying on its side next to my pillow. I killed it hours ago, and really wish that I had more, but I'm not going to risk leaving. I can tell that it is still light outside, but I have been watching the shadow from the window sill behind me slowly creep across the opposite wall. It must be past noon at this point. Evan could be here any minute.

I try not to think about my family or anyone else that I will be letting down by using again. I'm going to try my hardest to make this a onetime deal, and then perhaps I can try again to stay clean for good. I anticipated it being very hard for me to begin with, and never thought I'd even make it this far. There is some credit there to be had, which I know that I am going to ruin. I just can't go any longer without at least a small taste. Hopefully it doesn't do the same damage that I'm used to. Hopefully I can stop again before I go on another self-destructive rampage. Hopefully.

Hell

A small knock on the door snaps me out of my trance, and I am instantly on my feet. It has to be him. I open the door quickly and Evan is standing there, ready to go. I already have my smokes and cash in my pockets as I push in the lock on the door and shut it behind us. We are down the stairs and in the car within a minute – pulling away from the building in record speed. The journey has finally begun.

Trying to stay relaxed I throw in a tape that I had in my pocket and Evan smiles at the selection. We head toward the highway mixing in with the rush hour traffic from the day. Evan looks pretty chilled out, and I don't expect any weirdness from him, which is good. In a few short hours I'll have some relief from this madness and hopefully regain the ability to see things more clearly. I just need to feel normal for a little while, and then I'll be all set.

The highway is clogged with traffic and sets us back here and there, but not for any significant length of time. I watch the sun set as we move slowly through the exit into the city. Cars are everywhere and trying to stuff themselves all into the same place at once. Evan just nods along to the music and keeps his eyes forward at the red brake lights that grow brighter every few seconds. I try to stay relaxed in the passenger seat, and light another smoke. I'm going to need a new pack by the time we get back into town.

Evan is driving according to my direction as he has never been in this part of the city before. I suspect that he is going to be a little surprised at the way things look. Evan is one of the lucky people who has been sheltered from this area, and has only come down here for the normal consumer purposes. I hope that it doesn't freak him out too much.

The streets seem very dark tonight as we make our way through the tributaries that lead out to the edges of the city. These are the places where all of the action happens. This is where we all go when there is nowhere else to go. I love the streets here, but

I hate them just the same. I've already spent too much time here, and on a very intimate level. I've seen the gruesome and the ugly. I've seen what this place produces and churns out on a daily basis. The car jackings, the shootings, the gang activity, the drug deals. All the ugliness in the world can be found right here. With enough searching around you can get whatever you want – no matter how exotic. If you know the right people, and the right places – you can get your hands on anything. I've seen it done. I've utilized the services well, and can survive out here if need be. This is a place that I'm familiar with, and feel safe for the most part. The crazy people in the asylums are never afraid of the other crazy people there – they are afraid of everyone on the outside. It's the same for me when I'm here. I belong, and therefore am not afraid. I'll take what comes, and at least it makes sense. That's pretty much the only thing I ever ask for anyways – sense. That's it.

Evan takes another instructed turn and we start getting closer to the tattered house. My heart rate starts to increase and I remind myself to stay calm. It's been so long since I have been here that the excitement is hard to contain. I can't wait to get out of the car and make my way to the front door. The broken concrete slabs that make up the walk way have missed my footsteps these last few months. I'll be thrilled to feel them once again under my feet. My leg starts to shake and I stabilize it immediately, Evan doesn't even notice.

"Alright man, here's the deal. You're going to park up past that yield sign and in front of the church. I'm going to go to the spot on foot from there, you'll be able to see me from the car, but it's best not to park right in front of the house – trust me."

Evan doesn't even think about protesting, and is concentrating hard on not being affected by our surroundings. I can tell that he's uncomfortable about where we are and what we are doing, but he's trying to hide it the best he can. I don't think he expected it to really be this way. I can understand that to some extent, because people have a tendency to exaggerate about pretty much everything. By the serious look on his face it seems as though I haven't exaggerated enough. He was not prepared for this, but it's too late to change anything now, and he was the one who insisted. I try not to feel bad as the car finally comes to a stop.

"Give me a minute" I say to Evan, who simply nods and stares back out the windshield. Sitting there in the car I feel like I'm on fire. I can't wait to get this over with and have my hands on the dope once and for all. It has been so incredibly long since I have come here, and it seems like a century since I last used. Calm, calm, calm. I have to stay calm in order to do this correctly. I have to focus and fall back into the old routine, just for a few minutes. I know that it's still all sitting there inside of me – it should be easy to conjure up.

"Wait. Right. Here." I shut the door quietly behind me and head out toward the house. It's so quiet tonight that I can hear individual drops of water from the gutters attached to nearby houses. I continue walking down the uneven sidewalk with my eyes forward and my head down. I don't like it when things are this quiet – usually there's a reason for stillness. Focus.

I open the little gate at the edge of the yard and make my way up the walkway toward the front door. Before I can even do anything the door opens and I am motioned inside by a large Mexican man. I already don't like this.

"C'mon, c'mon...get in here fast." The man whispers to me. I recognize him, and I think he recognizes me too. He shuts the door behind us and peeks back out through a side window. He's looking for someone, or making sure that nobody is coming, I can't tell which. I've never actually been inside this house before, and my curiosity is killing me, but I do my best to not look around too much. I don't want to do anything too suspicious, especially under whatever circumstances these might be.

While staying low in front of the window he looks at me with an inquiring face. I toss him some cash and tell him the usual, and he reaches down with his right hand and picks up a packet. He throws it to me and looks back out the window. I really don't understand what is going on here, and then I notice the other man a few feet away aiming a rifle out of another window that also faces the street. Fuck. Of all the nights in the world I had to end up here tonight. You have got to be kidding me.

I quickly reach down and tuck the packet into my sock anticipating that the next few minutes are going to suck. I have no way to get in touch with Evan, and hopefully he's smart enough to stay clear when all hell breaks loose. This obviously isn't going to be a situation with police, because I doubt that there would be a gunman ready to take them all out. This is a defensive stance, which means that the shit storm is about to rain down on us at any time. Trying to see it before it comes is the only thing that we can hope for, and there's no way I'm going back out that front door any time soon.

"GET DOWN!!!!!" The Mexican man screams, and in an instant I am on the floor covering my head with my hands. The bullets shred through the wooden slats that protect us from the outside. Glass shatters all around me as bullets hit things in the house. Pictures hanging on the walls behind me shatter and explode into a million pieces. The man holding the rifle takes a bullet in the chest, but not before getting off a bunch of rounds. The entire house is filled with smoke and dust in an instant and then suddenly all is quiet. A faint screeching of tires can be heard a block or so away as everything in the room continues to settle. I check myself for blood even though I feel no pain, and find nothing thankfully. The Mexican man stands up and brushes some debris off of his shirt, but he seems unhurt as well.

"There's a door that leads to the backyard, you're welcome to use it, man." He says to me, almost completely unaffected by the assault that just took place. I watch him retrieve the rifle that is lying on the floor as I make my way toward the back of the house.

Hell

My legs feel like the insides of them have been replaced with soup. I fight back vomit as I make my way to the door. This isn't the first time that I have been shot at, but it still shakes me up just as much for some reason. It's not a good feeling. My first experience with guns was very up close and personal, and way worse than this one, but it's not something that I see myself getting used to anytime soon.

Once I am outside I can't tell if I feel better or more vulnerable. I really need to get out of this part of town, and I don't feel very safe doing so on foot anymore. Any association with this house could bring me down. That's assuming that I don't get jumped for some other reason that I don't foresee. I need to be careful making my exit, and have to do my best to stay out of view. The darkness is extremely helpful, but these people are very watchful and observant, which makes the task that much harder. Sneaking away from a house in the suburbs couldn't be easier. Getting away with shit out here is another story, once these people become you're enemies – you're fucked.

I stay in the shadows whenever I can, and use them to traverse from yard to yard. Dogs are also very bad around here, as most people use them for protection. I scan each yard carefully for any of the tell tale signs before entering, and when I do find one, I make my way carefully around it.

I successfully get back to the rear parking lot of the church and can't wait to be driving away from this place. I hope that Evan kept his cool during the whole episode. As I approach the front of the church I have a vision of his car with all of the windows shot out – my stomach knots up with a force that almost pushes me to the ground. I shake the image out of my head and come from around the side of the building. My stomach knots up again, but in a different way this time. Evan's car is nowhere to be found.

87. Stranded

duck back behind the church again so that I can get out of view as quickly as possible. I was not expecting Evan to be gone, and have no clue what to do. I'm in the middle of the ghetto and have no choice but to battle my way out on foot. I couldn't be less thrilled. I scored the dope, but with great cost. I have no way to get in touch with Evan, but I'm definitely not going to hang around here hoping that he'll return. Obviously he got freaked out and hit the road, I'm guessing that he just got back on the highway and is heading back home. He knew that when he left he would have no way to find me again, so I have to just assume he's gone for good. Time for plan B I guess.

I move through the neighborhood the same way that I did when I left the spot – analyzing each backyard before creeping through the shadows to the next one. Eventually I'll end up at a street corner and slightly less dangerous surroundings with each block that I pass. Once I get to safer ground I'll formulate my next move, but for now I have to focus on staying hidden. There are all kinds of bad shit going on out here tonight, and I have already been way too close to it. I don't want to get caught in the middle of anything else.

The ground is wet from rain that has accumulated over the past couple of days. By the time I get to blacktop again my shoes are completely soaked through with water and mud. Slopping through people's backyards will do that. I scramble through my pockets looking for loose change of any kind, or a dollar bill perhaps. I need to use a phone in order to get the fuck out of here. The only person that even knew I was here was Evan. My only option is to call my brother, but I need to have a logical explanation worked out in my head first. He's not going to be happy that I'm here, and his suspicions are going to be raised immediately. I find a one dollar bill in my pocket and head toward the street filled with stores to find a place that will break it for me. I need change for a payphone, and this task sucks sometimes. Some places won't open their register for you unless you buy something – its bullshit. Other stores seem to have no problem at all giving you change; it's just a matter of luck really.

I walk into the first gas station that I see and am immediately denied my request. Here we go. This is going to be fun, hopping from store to store just to get my hands on four quarters. I don't understand why some things have to be so fucking hard to execute. My patience is not what it used to be when it comes to things like this, and I'm really doing my best to keep it together. This night has been nothing but a fight since the minute I got out of Evan's car – I guess I should expect things to stay that way.

I finally catch a break by the time I reach a donut chain and manage to get my hands on some change. Conveniently there's a payphone right outside, and I am located at the corner of a very busy intersection right near the highway. I glance at the clock as I walk toward the payphone – 9:30pm already. Time flies when you're being shot at.

I really hope that my brother picks up the phone as I anxiously listen to it ring over and over. Finally he picks up, and answers in a strange suspicious tone.

"It's me. Listen, I need your help. I'm in a bit of a jam and need you to come get me." I say to him in my most sincere voice.

"No problem, where are you?" He asks.

"Well Evan needed to go to the mall down here in the city and he wanted me to go with him, but we got split up. I looked all over for him and finally decided to wait for him by the car, but when I got out to it he was gone. I have no clue why he decided to leave, but he's totally gone, I've been looking for him for hours." I answer, trying my best to be convincing. I don't even believe the bullshit that is coming out of my mouth, but I really hope he finds some thread of truth in my ridiculous story. I tell him which donut joint I'm at, and he agrees to shoot down and pick me up. I wait patiently on the corner and light up a cigarette.

At this point my nerves are shot. I have forgotten about the heroin stuck to my leg on the inside of my sock. The hell I went through to get it was enough to completely take my mind off of it. I'm more aware of things now than I was during the car ride down. The drive-by certainly shook me up a bit, brought me to my senses even. I feel differently than I did the other night at work when I was completely losing my mind. I'm still excited about taking this next hit, but I'm not as anxious for it – I'll be able to wait a day if need be. I have to eventually find Evan. I could use the remaining change that I have to give him a call, as he should be home by now, but I better just wait until I get back home first. The last thing I need to do is have something happen that would require me to make another call, and not have any money left to do so. I'm not going to make another move until I have to – just in case.

My brother knows the urgency of getting me out of here and therefore didn't think twice about dropping everything to come get me. I feel bad about this, because I don't want to exploit that quality within him. In reality I'm doing just that though. I am stuck in this shithole on my own accord. I explicitly came down here to score, and I am using my brother's hospitality, and fear of anything happening to me, in order to get back home. None of it sits right with me, but I don't really have a choice at this point. I always end up failing in the long run – give me enough time and I'm guaranteed to fuck things up. I still hope that at some point everyone who I care about will find a way to forgive me, even if it's just for being the person that I am. I never mean anybody any harm at all, and wish that I was hurting only myself with the choices that I make. That's the only thing that I want from everyone – forgiveness. I feel so bad when

Stranded

I think about all the things that I have done, and right now I'm really feeling like a loser. I made all of these problems for myself tonight, and I couldn't even get out of it all on my own. I was forced to call for help – I shouldn't be doing this shit anymore. I'm going to do whatever I have to in the future never to return to this place. My time here is up.

I am almost out of smokes when I see my brother's car pulling into the parking lot. A giant wave of relief washes over me as I make my way to the passenger side. My brother takes a good look at me when I get in the car, and apparently I pass the initial inspection because he gives me a little smile. I ask him to hook me up with a pack of smokes and we pull into one of the gas stations that I tried to get change from an hour or so earlier. If I didn't want to smoke another one so badly I would have told him to go somewhere else, but I just decide to roll with it. There's no need to actually make things more difficult than they already are.

The ride home was actually somewhat fun for me. My brother showed me a new album that he just got, which he thought that I'd like. He thought right. We listened to it the entire ride home, which was fast due to the lack of traffic on the highway. Traveling at night is usually so nice and peaceful; I had forgotten what it was like. I finally feel like I'm able to relax as we get further and further away from the diseased city. I usually feel safe when I'm in my brother's car anyway for some reason, which is odd because sometimes he drives a little crazy. I can't wait to get back to my room, and find myself getting anxious as we get closer. I usually can't wait to get away from it, but this night has certainly taken its toll on me. I'm even looking forward to sleeping.

I tell my brother to swing by the store tomorrow during the day so I can hook him up with twenty bucks for gas money. He waves his hand at me but says that he'll stop in when he gets out of work. I walk over to the payphone in front of my building before going upstairs and pull out the rest of the change from my pocket. Evan's house phone rings a few times and he picks up without answering.

"Hey – it's me man, chill out I'm home." I say right away.

"What the fuck happened down there? I had no idea what to do so I just hit it – I thought you were dead and that I was somehow going to be next. I'm really sorry man, Christ I'm glad you made it back. How did you-"

"Don't worry about it – pick me up from work tomorrow night and we'll go up to your place, for now just relax...everything is fine." I hang up the phone and head in through the front door of my building.

88. Last Day

I spent the day happy to be back in my room, and happy to still be alive. The reality of last night finally hit me this morning and I can't stop thinking about how lucky I was to have not gotten hit. I was also lucky to have gotten out of there on foot with nothing else happening. I need to stay away from that place as much as possible, and hopefully that was my last time going there for quite awhile.

I'm looking forward to going to Evan's tonight, and can't wait to finally feel that rush again. It seems like it has been a lifetime since I last felt it. I just have to make it through these next few hours. I've made it this far already, this one last stretch is nothing in comparison. I pack up my shit and head out to the street so that I'm not late for work. They have already talked to me about not showing up the other day, but believed that I was deathly ill and throwing up all over the place. Sometimes there are huge advantages to actually not owning a phone.

My shift is always busiest when I first get there, because that's when people are rushing around to get home. Things usually taper down a bit as the night moves on, which is nice, but for the most part it stays pretty steady. I have already made the decision to call Nikki as soon as things die down and I can comfortably use the phone without interruption. I don't expect the call to go very well, but I need to at least keep trying. I just need her to actually listen to me. I haven't talked to her for a few days, so I'm hoping that perhaps she'll have thought about things further. We'll see.

The little bell attached to the door hinge keeps ringing every few minutes, which means that someone has either just walked in or left the store. The bell hits the door differently when someone comes in, so I always know when it means more work for me. Its music to my ears when I hear it go off as somebody exits, because that means there's one less person to deal with. Once that last person is out of the store a mad dash to the back ensues so that I can get a phone call started as quickly as possible, in order to maximize the small window of non-interruption. That's exactly what I do as I hear the bell make its last funny little jingle.

Phone in hand – Nikki's number dialed.

"Hello?" She answers

"Hey....I was just hoping that you'd hear me out again." I say in a pleading tone.

"No. Why do you insist on doing this all over again? I already told you that I'm not having another child – I can't even manage to see the one that I already have, there's no way that I'm going to do that all over again. No way." She yells at me immediately.

"Seriously...listen...I just need-"I hear a loud click ring out through the receiver, like someone just cut the cord to the line outside. She must have slammed the phone down with force. I hope that it broke at least. Fuck. I don't even bother calling her back, there's no point, at least not tonight. She obviously is not in a rational state, or at least not rational enough to speak to me about this. I'll try again tomorrow, but I am quickly losing all hope of actually getting anywhere. I didn't think that I had any hope left to lose, but apparently I do – either that or I'm just plain stupid. I don't know. I can't give up just like that though, and I won't until the deed is actually done, which will then leave me no choice. Until then however, I have to do what I can to fight it. I just hate every minute of it.

The thousand year old cow bell jingles letting me know that a new customer has entered the store. The abrupt ending of the phone call couldn't have had better timing. They just want a pack of smokes and four different two dollar scratch tickets. I perform the tasks with my mind still pondering everything else. I have heroin. I can't stop telling myself that, and I can't wait to inject it into my body once again. Whenever I think about it for more than thirty seconds I get shaky with excitement. It's been way too long.

I hear the cowbell again and look up toward the door – my brother is here. I motion him to meet me out near the back door of the store. He turns around and leaves instantly. I grab a couple of packs of smokes and head toward the back. He's there waiting for me when I open the door. I light up a smoke and toss him a fresh pack along with the twenty dollars I promised him for gas. I can tell that he's looking me over for signs of possible heroin use. His suspicions about last night are dead on, but I still haven't given any clear proof to validate any of them.

I want to tell him about the Nikki situation, but I still can't bring myself to talk about it. It feels wrong to not tell him though, and even more wrong to not hear his input on the matter. I decide to give him a taste.

"There's some fucked up shit going on between Nikki and I. I can't go into detail right now about it, but I just wanted you to know that shit isn't going very well."

My brother nods his head, and doesn't even further question me. He's gotten very patient with situations like this, and doesn't bother wasting his time unless he actually thinks he's going to get somewhere. It obvious that I'm not going to go any further with it, so he absorbs what I tell him, and lets it go. At least I have given him a little bit of preparation so that he knows something is coming. He knows that it's something significant, or I never would have even mentioned it. He'll wait until I want to discuss it further. The conversation shifts and he moves on to the next subject that is still on the table.

"My friend thinks that there's a room open in the house that he lives at. I'm going to hunt him down tonight and find out – see when it's available and confirm the price on it." My brother tells me.

"Evan is picking me up tonight at midnight, and I'm going to stay at his place, so if you find anything out before then hit me up here. Otherwise I'll just hook up with you tomorrow sometime." I reply. I watch two cars pull into the parking lot at the same time and realize that my little party is over – time to go back to work.

"I'll talk to you later then." Our hands touch for a moment, and I'm back in the store. Smokes, smokes, lottery tickets, gas, smokes, gas, tickets, coffee, smokes, gas, gas, lottery tickets. This goes on for hours and hours and hours. The rest of the products here on the shelves might as well be destroyed and never reordered – they are not wanted by these people. One by one they come and go – each with their own weird story dragging behind them as they move through the motions of their lives. I can't wait to leave tonight. I need what is waiting for me.

The phone out back rings and I realize that it's getting late. I pick it up and my brother is on the other end.

"My friend is going to double check with his landlord tomorrow about the room, so I'll know more then, but at least the ball is rolling." He says to me.

"Thanks man, that's cool." I reply

"Are you sure you're ok?" He asks me. I hesitate before answering, not sure what to say exactly.

"Yeah" I finally lie. We hang up and I walk back out to the register. The clock says 11:30pm, not much longer now. The walls of the store keep slowly moving in closer to me all at the same time in unison, and then they drift back to their original places. This has been going on for the last couple of hours at least. My mind has started occupying itself with strange imagery in order to get me through the night. It has been my coping mechanism for dealing with the time. The time that never really seems to get anywhere as I robotically hit the colored buttons on the register. The time that laughs at me with every ticking sound it makes, every silent movement of the minute hand.

Last Day

I finish sweeping the floor – which wasn't very dirty to begin with, mostly because it's not raining out tonight. I can see Evan's head lights shining through the windows as he waits in the parking lot for me to come out. I put the broom away and throw the cash drawer from the register into the safe on the floor. My shift is up, and this place is closed. I flip the switch, turning off the lights, and head toward the front door with my keys in hand.

89. Asleep

I'm calm, for the most part, as we pull into Evan's driveway. I'm trying to stay on an even keel, and not get too excited. The dope is stashed away in my back pack which is sitting in between my legs in the passenger seat. The entire bag is glowing red and hot to the touch. It makes me nervous even to pick it up, but it's time to go inside.

Evan seems pretty collected, which is good, but there's a little bit of apprehension in his eyes that I am picking up on. I think he's nervous, perhaps because it has been so long since his last hit. The anticipation alone might be messing with his head; I know it's doing a number on mine. I wonder what his thoughts are right now in this exact moment. I wish I could listen in for just a minute or so in order to compare them with mine.

I'm finding it hard to focus as we get to the bottom of the stairs. Evan takes off his jacket and tosses it on the chair in the corner – I do the same. I set the back pack down in front of me and stare at it for a few seconds before I notice music suddenly filling the room. That's much better. Now that the tension has been lifted a bit, I can concentrate on everything that is about to transpire. I know that I shouldn't be doing this, but I feel as though I need to. I need to in order to survive for as long as I possibly can. I can't deal with the realities of my life anymore. I've literally gotten to the point where I can't face anything. I can't handle the ugliness that surrounds me, and I need the solace that only heroin can provide.

The zipper on my bag is loud and drowns out all sound in the room as I open the back pack. Everything inside is ready to go. I've been through hell and back to get my hands on this shit, and there isn't a force powerful enough that could keep me from using tonight. The works are waiting and zipped up in a small pouch that I came across along the way somewhere. I miss the wooden box, but at the same time – I don't. I have a lot of memories surrounding that box, but most of the ones I remember are bad. It's funny how it always works out that way – the good memories get pushed aside so easily, and we focus on the bad ones more. Maybe it's because the bad memories hurt, and pain leaves a mark that isn't easily ignored. The wooden box is a symbol of that, and I'm glad I don't have it with me tonight.

I set everything down on the little table in the middle of the room; Evan walks over slowly and pulls out a chair. We are silent, but focused, and the ritual begins. My lighter burns proudly under the small metal cap as the concoction inside gently bubbles to completion. I draw the first needle full and set it aside for Evan. Preparing mine is difficult as my hands keep shaking, but eventually I get it just right. Now we're ready. This is what it all comes down to. Right here in this basement, all of the waiting in the world has come to a stop. My senses are freed and I am aware of everything in this instant. I smile and pick up Evan's dose slowly. His arm is laid out before me, and I send him on his way once again. His reaction reflects the potency, and I am on the brink of losing control. I need it – now.

The needle enters my vein perfectly, like there was no hiatus at all. Sweat beads up on my forehead as I get ready to take it all in. The mixture floats around in the clear tube and swirls with my blood – waiting. I watch it slowly disappear into my arm. My head disconnects from my body and floats away. The rush is incredible, and not quite anything that I have ever felt before. I can tell that the stuff is strong, and coupled with my recent vacation – it's really taking me for a ride. I can't seem to get a grip on myself, and then everything starts to fall apart.

My breathing is heavy, the heaviest I've ever felt it. I can't get a full breath no matter what I do. I have managed to get myself on the floor and up against Evan's bed, but my lungs will not fully expand. Trying not to panic I look around the room for

Standing Room Only

Evan. He's laying on the floor a few feet away writhing around in the grips of his own battle. What have I done?

I'm starting to become uneasy with every second that passes, because things aren't stabilizing – they're getting worse. My heart beat is firing off once every twenty seconds. My mouth feels like it has been filled with glue, which only makes gasping for air even more difficult. Every muscle in my body is flexing beyond my control and rendering me unable to move. Could this really be it? Could this really be the end?

My symptoms are growing stronger and I try to crawl toward Evan for help. I need to get his attention, but I'm not even sure if he's capable of doing anything. I keep trying to move across the floor, but I'm not getting very far, in fact I'm not really getting anywhere at all. All objects in the room are distorting before my eyes, and everything seems to be moving slowly, yet here I sit and wait. It's too late to do anything now. I'm in trouble. I feel no physical pain, except for the breathing, but I am scared out of my mind with what is happening. I don't want to die – but I'm going to.

A surge of vomit pushes me to the ground as all of the sounds in the room start to fade away. A beautiful silence has replaced everything, and I can feel the tears fall from my eyes. There are so many people that I want to see right now, and I know that I'll never see them again. The emotional pain has broken through the drug, and hurts more than anything else in the world. I'm not ready to go – but I don't have a choice.

My arms wrap around my knees and I brace myself for the final note. My mind is filled with all of the people I love – I'm going to have to rely on them to bring me over to the other side. There's no other way to deal with this. I am sorry for everything that I have ever done, and for every ounce of pain that I have caused each and every one of them. If only they could read my thoughts.

Asleep

There's no more fight left in me, and I relax against the floor. My body is shaking, but I can't feel the discomfort inside. I know what is happening, but am numb to its effects. I know that closing my eyes will only bring death quicker, but I let my lids shut slowly, taking one last look at the room. The blackness is calming as the world starts to fade away from me inch by colossal inch. Freedom is calling to me finally, and I can almost feel myself drifting away. A profound sense of safety has enveloped me – if only I could freeze this moment forever.

Dear Disease,

     Lament for the loss of my bitter tasting lover. I suppose I have to live without you for as long as I can manage. And all of the things that go along with you, the rituals, the schemes, the satisfaction of obtaining you when just this morning it seemed impossible. To feel once more the rush of your entrance into my body. It's not that I won't think about you, not one second goes by that I don't. You're always in my head, and in my dreams, that is, when you allow me to sleep. I'll remember the times we had, and try to live a productive life without you. Knowing that you're out there waiting for me always, while so many others fade away. So until we meet again....

~Jason Flanagan

Asleep

I would like to thank everyone in my life who gave me the strength and ability to write this book. The journey was intense, and at times I thought as though I'd never be able to finish. My family and friends have helped me get through this, even though some of you might not have heard it from my lips. Each little tidbit of support, no matter how small, was monumental throughout the process. Thank you all, once again, I hope that someday I can adequately repay each and every one of you.

~JL

Standing Room Only

www.ingramcontent.com/pod-product-compliance
Lightning Source LLC
Chambersburg PA
CBHW050445150626
46551CB00029B/1698